THE COMPREHENSIVE VIBRATIONAL HEALING GUIDE

Life Energy Healing Modalities, Flower Essences, Crystal Elixirs, Homeopathy & the Human Biofield

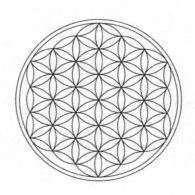

Other books by Maya Cointreau:

Gesturing to God
Mudras for Physical, Spiritual and Mental Well-being

The Healing Properties of Flowers
An Earth Lodge® Guide to Flower Essences

Natural Animal Healing
An Earth Lodge® Guide to Pet Wellness

Grounding & Clearing
Being Present in the New Age

Equine Herbs & Healing
An Earth Lodge® Guide to Horse Wellness

To The Temples
14 Meditations for Healing & Guidance

Also from Earth Lodge®:

Energy Healing for Animals & Their Owners
An Earth Lodge® Guide to Pet Wellness

THE COMPREHENSIVE VIBRATIONAL HEALING GUIDE

Life Energy Healing Modalities,
Flower Essences, Crystal Elixirs,
Homeopathy & the Human Biofield

MAYA COINTREAU

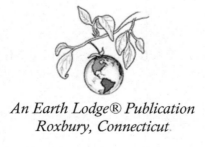

An Earth Lodge® Publication
Roxbury, Connecticut

For my children, bringers of light and joyful wisdom.
Shine on, little ones, shine on.

"We can starve as much from a lack of wonder as we can from a lack of food. If only for a little while, let us open our heart and see what glories unfold." – Ted Andrews

Table of Contents

Foreword

Have you ever read a book on the subject of vibrational healing and thought to yourself, "I want to do what they are talking about", only to put down the book and walk away because what you read just wasn't quite clear enough on the how-to?

This wonderful book will guide and direct you through the many modalities of vibrational healing. You will feel like Maya is sitting right there with you, talking to you on a personal level. She'll take you on your journey towards a new way of living life. Here she takes her personal experience to a new level and gets you started in vibrational healing.

As you begin to explore the beautiful world of flower essences and minerals you might wonder why you haven't explored this before. All I can say is that, you never picked up one of Maya's books. She makes it easy to relate to the material of whatever she is writing about. Her words will leave you feeling confident and self-empowered, ready to approach a world you might not have been able to before.

I have been in the field of energy healing since 1992 as a Polarity Therapy Practitioner. I have been working with Maya in the field of energy healing for ten years. I know who is just writing about this type of material and I know who lives what they are talking about. Maya lives what she talks about, and is sharing her wealth of information and insights with you. How blessed we are!

Kathy LaLonde, Polarity Therapy Practitioner

What are Vibrational Remedies?

We are all made of energy. Our bodies are actually a fantastic mixture of empty space, light-waves, and pure energy. All of it pulsating, dancing, mixing and twirling on sub-atomic levels which in turn fuel these powerhouses of possibility we call bodies. Everything we know here on earth, each thing we can touch, taste, and smell, these are also made of energy. The air, the furniture, the foods, the perfume, even the living. It's all just energy. Nothing more. Nothing less. Complex, yet simple.

Vibrational remedies are energy medicine. They are physical tools that heal and alter the energetic imprint contained within our physical body. The most well-known of these remedies in the West are probably homeopathy and reiki. However, there are many forms of vibrational remedies, including flower essences, Rife machines, bioenergetic medicine, and light therapy.

Some remedies seek to obliterate dis-ease by using its very own energy imprint to weaken it (homeopathics) or finding the specific frequency that will destroy it (Rife, bioenergetics). Others focus on strengthening the body and spirit so that the body can lift itself out of dis-ease (flower and crystal essences). All vibrational remedies shift our energy so that we can feel better. So that we can **be** better.

1

Everything has its own unique frequency. Atoms ripping through space and time to create what we hear, see, smell and touch. Even images and words have their own power, their own energy. They have frequencies that can affect the structure of water, literally imprinting it with their energetic signature. Studies have been conducted in many parts of the world that bear out this idea – Masaru Emoto's book "The True Power of Water: Healing and Discovering Ourselves" lists many examples. It is filled with both gorgeous and disturbing images of how our very thoughts can change the structure of water. The words "ugly" and "hate" create deformed ice crystals without structure, while words like "joy", "love" and "gratitude" can transform the same damaged water so that it will form crystals with the most intricate, breathtakingly beautiful crystalline symmetry, or even the image of the Buddha himself. Taping words or placing objects in water has been found to alter its energy signature, which in turn can have a beneficial impact upon the cellular structure of the body.

Vibrational remedies are about possibility. There is no can't, won't or shouldn't. It is one of the most hopeful and optimistic aspects of medicine, using light and love, the pure energies of Source which flows through all life on earth, to improve our condition. Those who have been bogged down by minds set in fear and doubt are quick to laugh at the ideas behind most vibrational medicine, but the beneficial effects clearly outweigh those of placebos. Rife machines are used extensively in hospitals and clinics throughout Eastern Europe, and Homeopathy has enjoyed countless documented successes in scientific trials. Throughout most of the world, homeopathy is accepted as regular medicine, and its derivatives are sold at pharmacies. Flower and crystal essences have also been the subject of many in-depth trials. In my own practice, we have used them with babies and animals and seen remarkable effects

– in other words, we have used them on beings that do not experience placebo effects. Either something works on a dog or a baby, or it does not. They do not expect that a splash of something in their food is designed to help them sleep through the night or stay calm during the day. Their energy merely shifts and flows, without them knowing why.

Vibrational remedies balance inharmonies on an emotional, physical and spiritual level. They may be used to heal the mind and ease bodily discomfort stemming from emotional or spiritual issues. Physical remedies made of water, alcohol, vinegar or sugars are considered safe for any age or size animal, whether human, horse, dog, cat or bird. Generally vibrational remedies are taken close together for acute situations or in times of extreme stress (15-30 minutes apart), or daily or weekly to trigger long-term change and healing.

Unlike conventional medicines, side-effects tend to be minimal with the use of vibrational remedies, although sometimes a "healing crisis" or "Herxheimer Reaction" may occur, wherein the subject initially feels worse as the therapy drives toxins from the body and re-aligns our polarity. This is a good sign to back off the remedy slightly, or to supplement your regime with complementary, supportive herbs or remedies. Bach's Rescue Remedy and Earth Lodge's Ease and Flow both have calming effects on the body and mind and are perfect for this sort of situation. The best vibrational healers have learned how best to avoid these sorts of reactions in their clients, preferring a gentle progression of healing rather than conducting an all-out war on the body.

How Do These Remedies Work with Our Bodies?

There are a variety of ways to explain the energy systems of the body. In Ayurveda and Kabbalah we have the chakras and the tree of life, in traditional Chinese medicine we have the meridians, and in polarity therapy we have the elements and the oval fields. Holistic healers talk about the aura, the merkaba, the energy body and light body as if they are all easily discerned and verifiable facts. Of course, this can be confusing.

What we do know, what has been proven through regular scientific method and observation, is that the body is energy and that this energy is measurable at a distance from the body. We know that our energy reacts with and affects the world around us. We know that not only does our body emit heat and sound through its electrical and physical activity, but *measurable* levels of light. We are all walking around giving off approximately 100 watts of infrared radiation, as well as hundreds of thousands of photons of every second – low-level light.

So can we really measure the aura? This thing called a biofield? Well, scientists have been using SQUID magnetometers for over 35 years to quantify the biomagnetic fields of humans. Scientists at MIT and other universities have verified that not only does each organ in the body emit a distinct, measurable field of energy, but also that energy healers and Qigong practitioners *emit the full spectrum of frequencies needed for cellular repair from their hands* when they are participating in active hands-on healing. Quantum physicists have seen that the mere act of a human observing an electron experiment from another room has an effect upon its outcome.

Scientists such as Reinhold Voll have measured the electrical status of meridians and acupuncture points and found that they do indeed have definite, measurable variations in frequency or flow. Furthermore, when an associated organ is debilitated or the person is in proximity to a harmful substance, readings will drop significantly. This research has been used to grow an entire field centered on the biofeedback one can receive from such instruments, allowing practitioners to easily determine whether a vitamin or food substance will actually benefit or harm a specific client.

The remedies in this book are all designed to balance or enhance the energy patterns in the body so that it can heal itself. All adults and children have stem cells in their body called "somatic stem cells" which are capable of renewing dying cells and regenerating entire organs from just a few cells. Yet most of humanity continues to sicken on a regular basis and our organs do not always regenerate themselves perfectly. We die. Why? Because our energetic blueprint becomes corrupted. We take medicine to heal ourselves, but modern allopathic medicine is not designed to recalibrate our blueprint, to balance our energy. Our cells can not heal themselves because we are, on an atomic level, distorted. This is where life energy healing modalities come in.

This is where the miracles begin.

Loving Life

Before you can begin to bring your body back into balance and facilitate a state of self-healing, you need to reawaken your mind-soul connection. It is not enough to simply live life. I want you to love life.

What's the difference?

When you are living life, you are going from task to task, moment to moment, without any real awareness of the process or the goal. Sometimes you are happy. Sometimes you are not. When things change, you worry. When things get better, you get excited. You try to do some things to help yourself and others, but mostly you are a passive member of humanity, reacting to circumstances as they occur and never quite feeling fulfilled or joyful. When you are loving life, you are L-I-V-I-N-G. You approach each moment with your eyes and your heart wide open. You are accepting of each new circumstance, and you are consistently approaching other people with compassion and seeking to understand and enjoy life to its fullest. You want to be a better person. You want to improve the life of all beings. You want to make the world a better place. Where you go, light shines.

Why does it matter?

When you are loving life, you are inviting your higher self, your oversoul, your infinite-I, your spark-of-god-self into your life. Your actions result in improvements for the highest good of all involved. You feel happier. You age more slowly, or not at all. Your health improves. Progress is made more easily at work and at home. People around you seem happier – when you smile, they smile. You are, indeed, making the world a better place.

When you are living life, you are not improving on anything. You are merely subsisting. You develop illnesses. You age. You fear. You cry. When you shout or glare, other people feel bad. You are, unfortunately, making the world a little bit worse. A little bit sadder. A little bit colder.

What can you do?

There are so many ways to begin loving life. It all starts with you. In your heart and in your mind. Sometimes, we are so not loving life that we need to begin with baby steps. Many vibrational remedies help open the mind to new solutions, making it easier to change gears and propel ourselves into higher realms of consciousness, or at least help us achieve a healthier emotional state.

Affirmations and **EFT** (Emotional Freedom Technique) both help to reprogram the mind and are great places to start. Affirmations are very, very easy to incorporate into your everyday life. Simply choose life-affirming statements and say them to yourself throughout the day: stick post-its on your mirror or your computer, in your car or on your lunch. Keep these statements positive, always confirming the best aspects you are seeking to encourage in your life.

Here are some examples of affirmations:

"I am happy and relaxed. I greet each new day with anticipation and enjoyment."

"I am surrounded by loving, caring people. I see friendly faces wherever I go."

"My food sustains my soul and body. I am nourished by healthy meals and a positive environment."

"My work fulfills me and is for the highest good of all. I enjoy going to the office each day and creating a better world. Every little thing I do makes a difference."

The wonderful thing about affirmations is that every time you say one of these statements, both your ego and your subconscious minds take note. You use your conscious mind to utter words, and your ego hears you. Your subconscious mind also notices that you are making these statements and proceeds to adjust your hormone levels and synchronize your heart and mind so that you will notice more of the positive aspects of life that are regularly occurring around you.

Meanwhile, each affirmation is like a prayer, too. The words you speak emerge as sound waves that literally go on forever. Every positive statement you utter creates a positive vibration that will emanate throughout the universe for all time. The same holds true for each negative statement. Which would you rather fill up the universe with? Which sort of frequencies would you rather surround your descendents with? These affirmations, these prayers, go out into the ethers and your higher self hears them. Your spirit guides hear them. Your ancestors and your gods hear them. All of source, all of creation, hears them. And the universe jumps to answer you, conspiring to co-create your most wonderful dreams with you.

EFT is similar to affirmations, except it also brings your body into agreement with your ego and your subconscious. In EFT, you tap on specific meridian points while you state your affirmations. Another difference is that you begin by stating your current negative statement. Below, I outline an EFT example, but I also suggest you check out the internet. There are a lot of great EFT instructional videos on YouTube – I find this the best way to really learn EFT.

How to do an EFT treatment:

While using the four fingers on your dominant hand to tap on the karate chop point, the side of your palm which your pinkie connects to, say the following three times, stating your physical or emotional pain as specifically as possible (this is statement called the "set-up"):

"Even though I _____, I completely love and accept myself."

Then tap on each of the following points in order, while saying a positive statement or simply "I love and accept myself"

- Top of the Head/Crown

- Inside of Eyebrow

- Side of eye

- Under eye

- Under nose on the philtrum

- Under your lip above your chin

- Collarbone

- Under the underarm

- Back to top of head.

Perhaps you've been feeling angry when you think about work. You could begin with the statement "Even though I am frustrated and angry at work, I completely love and accept myself" while you tap on your karate chop point.

Then you'd tap on each of the following points in order with the following statements, beginning with the most accessible or easy to accept statements of feelings first:

- Crown Chakra/Top of the Head, "I love and accept myself."

- Inside of Eyebrow, "I am comfortable in my office."

- Side of eye, "I like my co-workers."

- Under eye, "I enjoy my work."

- Under nose on the philtrum, "My work results in good for everyone."

- Under your lip above your chin, "It is fun finding new ways to agree and solving problems."

- Collarbone, "I am easy and go with the flow at work."

- Under the underarm, "I love what I do."

- Back to top of head. "I love and accept myself."

EFT works best when repeated often throughout the day. Get creative, and have fun with it.

Quiet your mind.

Another nice way to detox the mind and help the body heal itself is to incorporate meditation into your life. Even if you only meditate once a month, you will benefit. If you can meditate every day, so much the better.

A lot of people are scared to meditate, and think that they have to achieve great yogic states of consciousness to be successful. Not so! Real meditation is as easy as breathing and sitting. Sit down somewhere comfortable and just focus your eyes on a spot 3-6 feet in front of you. You can do this anywhere, anytime. Although it will work best if no one's trying to talk to you or get your attention. Sit and look, without any particular goal or intention. Pay attention to your breath out. Push it all out, deep from your diaphragm. Don't worry so much about breathing in – that will happen automatically. Just breathe out, and then let your body return to its natural state of being pure-breath filled. Thoughts will occur. When they do, just say to your self "thinking" or "there's a thought" and let it go. Don't judge, don't label. They are all just thoughts. No good ones, no bad ones. Just thoughts. Let them go, just like your breath. Breathe out, and then let the air flow back in. Breathe out, then in. Push toxins out, good air returns. Push stale air out, good air returns.

11

This sort of meditation helps your body re-learn how to breathe properly, something that most of us forget as we develop attitudes of stress and worry. It also gives your mind some time off, free time, so that when you do decide to let all those thoughts back in you can look at them with a fresh set of mind-eyes.

Do what you love.

Remember to do the things you love. Eat the food you like. Choose activities that make you happy. Be clear – an activity that dulls the pain is not the same as an activity that brings you joy.

If you are not enjoying what you are doing, it is not in vibrational alignment with the real you. When you are sad, it is because you are thinking thoughts that will not help you achieve what you are wanting. When you are happy, you are in full alignment with your higher self. You are filled with source energy. You are energized and flowing with all that is. You are at peace. You are joy-full.

Take time to do things for yourself, even if it's just two minutes a day. Even if it's just a matter of buying your favorite cheese at the market as a treat. It is important, on the path of healing, to make sure that you feel nurtured. It is important to make yourself comfortable and at ease. Only then can your body begin to believe that you want to help it, not use it until it breaks. Life feels best when our body, mind and spirit are all working in tandem, in agreement. When you ignore one to nurture the others, you will suffer as a whole. All three must be sustained and appreciated for your physical life on earth to reach its full potential.

When we are angry or sad, those emotions become stored in our energetic imprints, and eventually manifest as dis-eases in our physical bodies. Luckily we live in a physical plane that incorporates the concept of "Time" and so we have a buffer of time between our thoughts and when they manifest -- we have time to remedy negative thought imprints before they manifest in our bodies or our lives. Take steps to love yourself and the life you lead, and you will begin to improve your reality in ways you may not even have dreamed of.

Navigating the Human Biofield

When you begin any sort of work in the alternative medicine field, pretty soon you will begin to come across terms that you might not be familiar with. Chakras. Meridians. Oval Fields. Energy Centers. Wheels of light. Tree of life. Caduceus.

Be prepared. When you mention to your yoga teacher that you are feeling a little nausea, she might respond that your third chakra is "out of whack" and could use some clearing work. Huh? What?!

Don't worry. It's not all that complicated. Just a quick little chapter and we'll have you spinning wheels of light with the best of them.

Just as your physical body has organs, arteries and veins, your energy of your biofield flows in distinguishable patterns. In India, they describe this with the Tree of Life and Chakras. In China and Japan, energy flow works with the meridians. In Polarity therapy, there are oval fields, chakras, and energy currents. Everything works together to explain the way that energy flows through your body, keeping balance and maintaining optimum levels of health and energy.

Wheels of Light

Let's begin with the chakras. The word chakra is derived from ancient Sanskrit, and means, simply, a point of energy or power. You have many chakras, or energy centers, in your body. You have them in your feet and hands, your legs and arms, above and below and throughout your body. There are seven primary chakras that are referred to most often. The largest chakras are known both by their location and by numbers denoting their order of ascent on the body. The higher upwards you travel, the higher the number of the chakra. They are generally described as spinning wheels or vortices of light.

If your chakras are spinning well, they are "open, and you are healthy. When a chakra slows down or stops spinning, it is described as "closed" or "blocked". Energy in the biofield needs to flow clearly and regularly in a circuit. If part of the field is blocked, other places in the biofield will eventually suffer, much like the heart suffers when an artery is clogged. First, the chakras closest to the blockage will be affected, as well as the physical organs related to that chakra. Eventually, the entire system suffers.

First Chakra (Root Chakra)

At the base of your spine, deep within your pelvic area, the root chakra is the center of your intent to live. It is primal, sexual, survival energy. It governs your immortality and fuels your ability to ground and collect energy from the Earth (we'll talk more about earth and the other elements in the next chapter). Your root chakra is what determines your final physical manifestation here on our planet, it is what keeps you safe, what shields you from disease and physical harm. When it

15

is damaged, your life-force is endangered. It is associated with the colors red, black and brown, earthy tones. It affects the legs, bones, reproductive system, feet, and large intestine.

Second Chakra (Sacral Chakra)

Here in your lower abdomen is your intent to feel with all your senses, to experience your emotions and all aspects of your being: your subconscious and unconscious as well as your ego, your non-physical and dream selves, as well as that which is rooted in the physical. It is associated with the flowing energy of water. An underdeveloped intent to feel limits your sensitivity, and can be linked with your intent to live. The more feeling you are, the better you may perceive imbalances in your non-physical self, and repair the problem before it manifests in the physical. Second chakra issues generally pertain to your tribe, or community, and your perceived place within it, as well as issues of security and safety. It is associated with the color orange, and rules the lower back, genitals, hips and small intestine.

Third Chakra (Solar Chakra)

In your solar plexus, your third chakra houses your intent to protect, involving the ability to protect yourself through the creation of positive boundaries. Issues of ego and instability crop up here, as this chakra houses your personal power and ambitions. The third chakra carries fire energy, and is the center of your will and direction. It is here that Joy is needed to feed the soul, and so this chakra is associated with the color yellow or light green. Indigestion is a common symptom of unbalance in the third chakra.

Fourth Chakra (Heart Chakra)

In the middle of your chest at heart level is your fourth chakra, housing your intent to love and accessing unconditional love. Unconditional love manifests in the world as a compassionate flow of energy from your heart chakra. When this happens, love and compassion bless all of creation with the love from Spirit, and you are open to receive unconditional love yourself. This chakra is associated with both pink and green, pink for love and green for healing.

It is governed by air energy, the energy of movement. Problems of the lungs and heart are symptoms of its imbalance. In the past, the lower and upper chakras used to blend predominantly in the third chakra, and it was here that people would experience disconnection to their upper halves, but as humanity opens to unconditional love on mass levels, we are becoming centered in our heart chakras, and experiencing splits more and more in our throat chakra. Get ready to say hello to an increased prevalence of flus and allergies, and a decrease in unstable relationships, fear and anger on a global scale. These "splits" result from imbalances between our spirit, beliefs and ideals, and our physical, ego/earth-driven selves, and are best healed through an open heart.

Fifth Chakra (Throat Chakra)

Your fifth chakra is centered above your clavicle bone in your throat, and houses your intent to create, harnessing the flow of energy from Spirit and allowing you to manifest your dreams. The spiritual element of ether in your body is housed here, and feeds the other elements in your body. If your will is not flowing, your ability to dream and manifest is likewise impaired. The intent to create helps you bring your creative desires into physical being and is associated with clear, bright blue. Communication or informational related issues often manifest as sore throats or laryngitis, and can even affect the teeth and sinuses. Help the client identify what they would like to say, and speak their truth. It is generally associated with the color blue or turquoise.

Sixth Chakra (Third-Eye Chakra)

At your third eye, located about an inch above the bridge of your nose between your eyebrows, a few inches back in the middle of your brain, is your sixth chakra. This is your highest creative energy center, where your spirit meets your creative focus. Here is your intent to see. When you *Intend to See* you see the true reality of the universe, and the illusions of mass consciousness fade away. You will see your way clearly, and things will tend to fall into place. It is associated with the color violet or indigo. Blockages here can manifest as headaches, eye strain, sleep disturbances, or ear infections.

Seventh Chakra (Crown Chakra)

Your seventh chakra is located in the crown of your head towards the back where your soft spot was as an infant, and is where you have the intent to receive wisdom and evolve from your higher self and Spirit. It is place of pure potential. When this center is impaired, it is more difficult to receive the correct information you need to maintain a high vibration and stay on the path of evolution. It is linked with the color white, and is where you receive Qi from the universe. Crown chakra issues general manifest as mental disturbances, confusing thoughts, and apathy.

The Meridians

Meridians are Qi pathways in the body. They allow the energy in your biofield to flow from organ to organ, muscle to muscle, in a regulated, cohesive manner. Each meridian, like any line, is made up of an infinite number of points. Many of these points refer to specific organs or places in your body – just as each meridian regulates the flow of energy in specific areas of the system. When a point is blocked, the qi becomes stagnant or blocked, and illness may present in the body. According to Traditional Chinese Medicine, gentle palpation of specific points can often initiate movement and flow. Likewise, specific herbs and remedies are used to awaken the energy.

There are 20 primary meridians and close to 650 acupuncture points used in traditional meridian therapies such as acupressure and acupuncture. Reflexology is a more accessible derivative of this science, and focuses on the points in the feet which have correspondences throughout the body.

Oval Fields, the Tree of Life and the Caduceus

The Tree of Life is well known throughout the world as a creation story. It is also used in Ayurveda and the Kabbalah to represent the human biofield. Source energy is pictured spiraling down the staff of life, the caduceus, from the top in mirror waves, winding back and forth like two snakes in an image that reminds many people of DNA.

At the top, or head, we have Source energy as it enters the body. The staff itself represents the energetic core of the body, the spinal cord and the Central Nervous System. It is the neutral core or pole of the body, and holds the blueprint for physical form. Where the energy begins in the head and aura, the poles are reversed, with the masculine on the left side and the feminine on the right. As it crosses down into the body, the right side of the body is generally considered masculine, while the left side is feminine. The right is positive, yang, stimulating, expansive, restless and conscious. Paternal issues tend to manifest on the right side of the body. The left side is negative, receiving, contractive, dreamy and yin. Maternal issues manifest here.

As the energy expands and flows downward in both its feminine and masculine, or negative and positive aspects, it crosses several times, forming the oval fields as it travels down through the body. Each of these fields is related to a different element, a different energy, and corresponds to a different element governing part of the creation of physical life The oval fields are used to describe the quality of movement of energy through them, while the chakras refer to the quality of energy emanating from their centers.

The oval fields are easily found in the five main cavities in the body, the head (fire), throat (ether), the chest (air), abdomen (earth) and pelvis (water). The first oval field in the head governs thought, control and the fiery spark of creative direction. The second oval field in the throat has to do with the expression of spirit, sound and communication. The third oval field in the chest is about the movement of air in the body, circulation and life energy. The fourth oval field in the abdomen governs the functions of sustenance, assimilation, metabolism and the processing of nourishing matter in body. The fifth oval field in the pelvic bowl governs elimination and fluid activities in the body.

As with the chakras and meridians, if one oval field is blocked or malfunctioning other areas of the body will also begin to suffer pain or dysfunction. Where the fields meet problems can most easily arise, causing congestion and stagnation.

Each of the aforementioned energy systems seek to describe one thing. Our biofield is alive. It is a complicated web of energy. No one part of our body is truly independent of another. Every cell works together with a group. The better our biofield is functioning, the healthier and happier we will feel. And the better we feel, the better life can be. Vibrational remedies target various aspects of the biofield so that energy can move and flow to where it's going.

About the Elements

If you work with vibrational medicine for any length of time, eventually you will encounter references to the elements. These do not refer to the elements of weather (although they are related) but rather to the elements within the body. The elements have their roots in the very birth of life energy modalities: vitalism. The concept of vitalism is central to most systems of indigenous healing, as well as newer biofield therapies: Ayurveda, Reiki, Shamanism, Traditional Chinese Medicine (TCM), and Polarity Therapy all work around the basic premise that the proper function of the body itself is contingent upon the healthy flow of a vital life force. You may call this vital force Qi, Prana or Source Energy.

Most systems that center on vitalism also discuss the importance of harmonizing the elements within the body. When the elements are out of balance meridians become blocked, agitated or sluggish; chakras shut down; biological functions suffer. In general, there are between 3 and 5 elements addressed by most systems – the most common relating to Earth, Water, Fire, Air, Ether/Spirit, and Metal. When one element suffers, another will try to overcompensate, creating disharmony and eventually dis-ease in the body.

There are many ways to work with the elements in the body. You might choose particular foods which correspond to the element you wish to support, certain colors, temperatures or textures.

There are entire books and modalities which discuss how to work with elements. If you find yourself very interested in working with the elements, I recommend studying Polarity Therapy, Traditional Chinese Medicine, Ayurveda or Wicca (an elemental, nature based religion). What follows now are some basic guidelines for those wishing to begin exploring their relationship with the elements.

Earth

Color: Red, Black, Brown

Governs: Structure, Generosity, Courage, Survival, Stress Response

Parts of the Body: Skeleton, Digestion, Knees, Coccyx, Adrenals, Neck

Imbalance manifests as: Joint Pain, Digestive problems, Osteoporosis, Stubbornness, Fear, Stress, Spaced out, ADD/ADHD, Parasites

Stones: Ruby, Carnelian, Onyx, Obsidian, Smoky Quartz

Food: Food that grows below ground, Meat, Red food

Taste: Sweet, Earthy

Direction: North

In nature: Soil, Ground, Plants, Animals, Mountains

Animals: Horses, Grazing Animals, Canines, Bears

Water

Color: Orange or Blue, depending on the system

Governs: Emotions, Sexuality, Creativity

Parts of the Body: Feet, Bladder, Pelvis, Sacrum, Shoulder Blades, Chest, Breasts, Reproductive and Immune systems

Imbalance manifests as: Damp, Sweat, Water weight, Cold, Reproductive issues, Sadness, Emotional imbalance, Fungal issues

Finger & Toe: Ring

Stones: Larimar, Pearl, Anhydrous Quartz, Orange Topaz, Amber

Food: Food that grows from ground level to two feet, Orange Food, Fish, Seaweed

Taste: Salty, like the ocean, or Wet

Direction: West

In nature: Oceans, Rivers, Lakes, Wells, Rain, Snow

Animals: Frogs, Fish, Turtles, Whales, Dolphins

Fire

Color: Yellow, Red or Orange, depending on the system

Governs: Personal Power, Expansion, Motivation

Parts of the Body: Thighs, Pancreas, Umbilicus, Liver, Solar Plexus, Eyes, Forehead

Imbalance manifests as: Fever, Anger, Resentment, Digestion issues, Dull eyes, Warts

Finger & Toe: Middle

Stones: Fire Agate, Opal, Citrine, Volcanic Rocks

Food: Food that grows two to six feet above ground, such as grains; Hot Spices; Yellow Food

Taste: Bitter, Spicy

Direction: South

In Nature: Lightning, Fire, Heat

Animals: Phoenix, Dragons, Lizards, Snakes, Salamanders, Felines

Air

Color: Blue, Yellow or Green, depending on the system

Governs: Desire, Motivation, Mental Support, Intellect

Parts of the Body: Ankles, Calves, Kidneys, Thymus, Shoulders, Circulation, Respiration, Nervous System, Immune System

Imbalance manifests as: Circulatory issues, Lethargy, Insomnia, Focus issues, OCD, Headaches, Gas

Finger & Toe: Index

Stones: Blue Topaz, Emerald, Moldavite, Indicolite, Chrysocolla, Selenite

Food: Food that grows more than six feet above ground, such as nuts and fruits; Green or Blue Food

Taste: Sour

Direction: East

In Nature: Air, Clouds, Thunder

Animals: Dragons, Pegasus, Griffin, Flying Birds, Butterflies, Dragonflies, Ladybugs, Bees

Ether

Color: Blue, Purple, White or Gold, depending on the system

Governs: Communication, Peace, Expansiveness

Parts of the Body: Joints, Body Cavities, Neck, Thyroid, Face, Hair, Skin

Imbalance manifests as: Grief, Dizziness, Accidents, Anxiety, Restriction, Low Self Confidence, Hearing Issues, Joint Pain

Finger & Toe: Thumb, Big Toe

Stones: Quartz, Imperial Topaz, Phenacite, Petalite, Amethyst, Apophyllite, Celestite

Food: Blue and black berries, Dark Grapes, Sprouts, very fresh and raw food; Blue or Purple Food

Taste: Variety

Direction: Center, Up

In Nature: Space, Gases, Caves

Animals: Fairies, Spirits, Angels, Unicorns

Touch-based Healing Therapies

Touch is one of the five senses. It is the first thing we know as babies in the womb, the feel of our own skin on our skin, the brush of the umbilical cord against our stomachs. When we are born, we are caught and held. As we grow, touch can be used to soothe us, to show love and support. A pat on the back, a hug or a kiss. It makes sense that touch would present itself as an important vehicle for healing.

We are electromagnetic beings, as we've seen. Our biofields interact with other people's bodies and biofields even before we touch them. Just being near another person can have an immense effect on their state of being. When you approach a person with the intent to heal, I believe that your biofield or aura is raised or pumped up, and interacts with the other person's life force with a beneficial effect.

So, what exactly are these touch therapies? The most well known touch therapies are Reiki, Polarity Therapy, and Healing or Therapeutic Touch. What each of these therapies has in common is that hands are laid on with the intent to direct and balance energy flow within the body. Many touch therapists and their clients report tingling or warm sensations while working, and believe that they may be directed by such sensations to the areas of the body that are the most in need of healing work. It is believed that through the active and consciously directed laying on of hands, that blockages or damages in the physical body and its energetic layers may be felt and recalibrated. This balancing effect then results in an improved sense of well-being on the part of the patient, and may be used to treat a variety of emotional, physical and spiritual imbalances.

It is difficult to quantify the benefits of touch therapies. Each healer has a varied approach and effect on his or her clientele, and placebos for the healing touch are problematic (one solution is to use a false hand, but studies have shown that pressure itself, even from a machine, can have a calming effect on animals and autistic patients. Nevertheless, research has been attempted by many scientific groups. Hands on healing has been found to reduce stress hormones and lower blood pressure and heart rates, while soothing subjects enough to offer possible pain relief and benefit depression. Some of the best hospitals in the United States have seen enough results to encourage them to offer reiki for palliative care – Yale, John Hopkins and Duke among them. I have spoken with many nurses who believe that the reiki training they have received enables them to offer greater benefits to their patients under their care, even if it's just to offer a quick reiki "boost" while they change their dressings.

Let's take a closer look at each of the touch therapies mentioned so far.

Reiki

Reiki is an energetic hands-on touch therapy which channels universal life energy, or Qi, through the hands of the practitioner and into the auric field and body of the client. Reiki combines traditional Japanese hands-on healing techniques with the meditative visions and teachings of Dr. Mikao Usui, born August 15th, 1865 in Gifu prefecture, Japan. The ability to channel this reiki energy (Rei means "universal spiritual wisdom" and ki means "life force") is passed from teacher to student through graded attunements. Each attunement works by opening the body's chakras and energy fields to better allow the transmission of these energies.

Because Reiki teaches that the practitioner is basically a "hollow tube", a simple channel of universal source energy, Reiki practitioners tend to feel better after treating their patients. The healing energies flow through them and around them when they activate their reiki centers. Since they themselves are not conducting the healing, but merely directing the beneficial energies, it is very rare for Reiki healers to pick up the symptoms of their patients – as can be common in many other forms of energetic healing.

There are three traditional levels of Reiki certifications (although some teachers have begun to split the final Master level into Reiki three and Reiki Master). These certifications are based on the attunements or openings they have received. Reiki One is the first level, and enables one to practice basic hand-on healing techniques with clarity and intent. Level Two brings in distance healing applications, so that the practitioner can transmit healing energy over long distances: beaming Reiki from one side of the room to the other, or even one country to another. The Reiki Master attunement activates body lightning, or kundalini, significantly amping up the healing energies within the practitioner. A Reiki Master also learns how to open others with Reiki attunements, and so the student becomes the teacher. When Reiki Master is split into two classes, Reiki Three and Reiki Master, the student receives the Master attunements in level three but does not learn how to pass attunements until Reiki Master.

Reiki has been shown in studies to reduce stress, induce relaxation and relieve pain in many forms. Can it heal the body? Anecdotal evidence is rampant. Although it remains to be proven, Reiki is believed by many to have profound healing potential. Certainly if one is relaxed the nervous system can quiet down, the immune system can function without interference and the body can began to heal itself in more effective ways. Try it and see!

External Qi Healing

Qigong is a Chinese system of energy manipulation over 2,500 years old. It combines breathwork, movement, and meditation to energize and balance the physical body while strengthening the spirit. Sometimes, other aids are brought into Qigong practice, such as herbal medicines or massage. External Qi Healing Therapy (EQH) is an aspect of Qigong which focuses on diagnosing energy imbalances in the body and directing the healing aspect of Qi, or life energy to restore balance and help the body heal itself. Remember the "Karate Kid" movie, when Mr. Miyagi partially healed Daniel's leg during the tournament? That was a perfect example of Qi Healing.

As Mr. Miyagi says in the movie, his lessons with Daniel are "not just karate only. Lesson for whole life. Whole life have a balance. Everything be better. Understand?" Qigong is related to martial arts as an exercise form. It also teaches balance and allows the practitioner to better align with universal life energy for health and vitality. The meditative techniques taught in EQH are believed to improve a healer's ability to sense and treat dis-ease.

In all aspects of Qigong practice, there is a major focus on proper breathing. Think you breathe the way your body intended? You probably don't. Most modern humans use shallow breaths from the lungs, barely using the diaphragm or abdomen muscles which are required for proper breathing. Babies breathe deeply. Animals breathe deeply. Our fast-paced lifestyle and poor postures contribute significantly to our "forgetting". The good news is the body can easily be retrained to breathe more deeply and healthfully, using simple breathing exercises for a few minutes every day. Our body wants to breathe at optimum levels, and given the slightest opportunity, it will. The easiest way to begin is to sit or stand with an erect posture, and put your hands on your diaphragm, the upper portion of your abdomen located below your ribs. Now breathe in and out, naturally. Does your chest rise and fall? Or does your diaphragm push your hand in and out? What you are wanting is more of the latter, and less of the former. Retrain your body to breathe properly by using the full range of your respiratory system, encouraging your diaphragm to work to its potential. Make sure you breathe in through your nose – breathing through your mouth alone can easily decrease the amount of oxygen you take in by 15% or more.

Polarity Therapy

Polarity Therapy is a system of touch therapy devised by Dr. Randolph Stone. Synthesizing his knowledge of Ayurveda, traditional Chinese medicine and chiropractic therapy, Dr. Stone created a powerful method of therapy which balances the positive and negative poles of the body and addresses a multitude of physical, mental or emotional imbalances through working with the five elements (Ether, Air, Fire, Water, Earth).

Each element, as discussed in the earlier chapter "About the Elements", corresponds to different areas of the body, affecting general health in that area, as well as impacting energy flow to other regions. For this reason, it is often suggested that students wanting to study Polarity Therapy first gain at least a basic knowledge and understanding of how the meridians and chakras work.

What can polarity therapy do for you? Most polarity clients report better focus, more comfort and enjoyment in daily life, and less stress. Polarity therapy can reboot and align the energy fields in your body, removing blockages or flow issues which may result in dis-ease or discomfort.

The elements, which correspond to different energy fields in the body, do not just relate to our physical bodies, either. They can greatly affect our mood or thought-process. If your fire element is out of whack, you might experience outbursts of anger. If your water element is deficient, you might be unable to relate to other people well or open up. A physical side effect might be kidney issues, incontinence or pain in your ring finger. And, of course, if one element is out of balance, it tends to affect other elements, too. Too much fire can cause a deficiency of air and water, too much air can lead to too much fire, and so on.

Sound complicated? There is a lot of information here than in some of the other touch systems, but once you get the hang of it, you'll see that Polarity work ties in very nicely with most other forms of vibrational healing, complementing and uplifting them.

Healing Touch

Healing Touch is, in practice and form, quite similar to Reiki, although it was developed independently and in an entirely different country. This simply demonstrates the interconnectedness of all beings, and how we are all born with an innate ability to heal and transform our realities. Healing Touch does not use symbols to the degree that reiki does, but it does introduce similar healing methods and energetic concepts while embracing a heart-based, loving energy as the source of all healing. It was created by Janet Mentgen, RN, BSN, an American nurse who was very sensitive to energy in the body. Over the years, she found that through opening her heart, her hands could naturally channel healing energy to her patients, decreasing pain and inflammation, alleviating stress and even closing wounds or energy leaks in the body. In 1989 she created the official certification program for the methodology, and in 1990 it was sponsored though the American Holistic Nurses Program.

Healing Touch has six practitioner degrees, and one must go through official channels of certification at each level. Healing Touch is wonderfully accessible to people in all walks of life, and has been especially well-received by fellow nurses and the rest of the medical community as a beneficial supplement to conventional healthcare.

Therapeutic touch

In the 1970s, Delores Krieger, PhD, RN, developed Therapeutic Touch (TT) with her mentor Dora Kunz, a natural healer. It is taught at over a hundred colleges in the United States and Canada, and has gained wide acceptance in the medical field as a supplemental healthcare treatment that brings relief and comfort to patients. Thirty percent of American hospitals offer TT to patients.

Although it was also created by a nurse and involves the word "touch", TT is quite different from the Healing Touch method. In fact, TT rarely involves any actual physical contact or touch. In practice, TT is actual a form of distance or aura healing. It works specifically with the biofield. The first part of a TT session consists of a quiet time wherein the practitioner stills and opens their mind to attune with the mind and body of the client. Then the hands are passed 2-6 inches above the body, diagnosing blockages and imbalances in the client's energy field. Finally, the hands are used "brush" the aura, gathering negative energy and flicking it away so that the energy can flow unimpeded in the body. This method is also taught as a part of most touch based therapies -- it is a very simple, yet effective way to diagnose issues in the biofield that are affecting the physical body, and it is a good start on the path towards healing and restoration.

Quantum Scanning

Quantum Scanning is an intuitive healing touch method that uses the polarized energy fields of the hands to initiate a healing flow of Qi throughout the body. It is very similar to Reiki or Healing Touch but requires no particular training or attunements. The healer begins by relaxing the mind and body, and connecting to both their own higher self and that of the client. The client generally stands facing the practitioner, although the work may be done in any position. The scanning begins by placing one hand on each foot and, scanning the subject with one hand and receiving the energy scanned through

35

the other hand. Energy is released in whatever manner is most practical or comfortable for the practitioner, although flicking or throwing motion is used most often. Then the hands are moved upwards to the knees, where the subject is again scanned and cleared of negative or vibrationally disharmonious. This continues up through the body to the hips, crown of the head and down the arms to the fingertips. Then the scanning is repeated on the back side of the client.

Life Energy Modalities
of the East

The nations of the eastern hemisphere of the Earth have long healing traditions, with written records of both herbal and energy healing systems going back thousands of years in many countries. The two most well-known eastern healing traditions in the United States are Ayurveda and Traditional Chinese Medicine (TCM). Other healing traditions worth noting are Traditional Vietnamese Medicine, or Dong Y, which intersects strongly with TCM; Kampo, from Japan; Won-Ki from South Korea; and traditional healing methods from Tibet.

Traditional Chinese Medicine
(also known as Dong Y or Eastern Medicine)

Traditional Chinese Medicine (TCM) combines body, mind and spirit into its treatment philosophy. TCM began over 2000 years ago, as documented in the Yellow Emperor's Inner Canon (ca. 100 BCE) and The Treatise on Cold Damage Disorders and Miscellaneous Illnesses (ca. 200 CE), and found in archeological evidence from the Shang Dynasty (ca. 1300-1000 BCE). The Canons of Problems (second century CE), The AB Canon of Acupuncture and Moxibustion (ca. 256-282 CE), and The Canon of the Pulse (ca. 280) all followed shortly after. As China expanded and interacted economically and culturally with nearby cultures, medical theories also grew and expanded, so throughout the centuries TCM also became closely related to Vietnamese, Korean and Japanese systems of healing. In the cases of Vietnam and Korea, both had long histories of medical tradition. Many texts and practices in Vietnam pre-date Chinese conquest, although the majority of what we consider traditional Vietnamese medical theory is intricately intertwined with that of China. Both cultures learned much from each other.

TCM looks at Qi energy as interplay of the five elements, flowing through and around the body. Earth, Air, Fire, Water and Metal are related to everything surrounding us, from the foods we eat to the colors we use in our clothing. Yin and yang, male and female, positive and negative aspects of the self and the environment play off of each other to further affect and harmonize Qi. Acupuncture, the practice of physically manipulating specific Qi points on the body using heat, smoke and/or fine needles, re-directs energy flows and removes blockages in the meridians ("rivers" of Qi which flow through the body). The practice of Feng Shui is also brought in to TCM, where it is believed that improper flow of Qi in the home or at work will also affect the health and integrity of the body.

Modern TCM combines herbalism, acupuncture, massage, diet, and exercise to treat the patient. Dis-ease is believed to originate from imbalances between the elements, poor energy flow in the meridians and even one's environment. It is a thorough and comprehensive system of healing based on vibrational principals. Of course, Western TCM differs very much from how TCM is practiced in China, where patients often receive acupuncture every day until a condition is resolved. Here in the United States, with health care and insurance costs increasing significantly every year, most patients can only afford to visit acupuncturist weekly or even less.

Fortunatelt, there is a new model of acupuncture being practiced in the United States called "community acupuncture", where services are rendered in less private conditions and can cost as little as $15 per treatment.

Another stumbling block to Eastern medicine in the US comes from our eating habits. In China, a meal is considered "good" if it is healthy. Foods are chosen more for their effect upon Qi than their taste. In the United States, foods are chosen primarily for how they affect our mood and palette. Health effects, beyond whether a food is organic or GMO, are rarely considered. Also, while the tenets of herbalism are widely accepted and integrated into nutritional practices in China, here in the West herbal apothecaries remain considered a relatively foreign and quaint idea. Despite long traditions of herbalism throughout Europe, it has been vilified so extensively by Western doctors over the last few hundred years that its widespread acceptance and resurgence remains seriously hampered.

Ayurveda

Ayurveda originated over 5,000 years ago in India, and means "The Science of Life" in Sanskrit. It is precisely that, a mind-body science of healing that integrates exercise, diet, meditation and herbalism to treat the energetic and spiritual components of the self affecting the physical body. Yoga is a part of the Ayurvedic system of healing.

Ayurvedic principles circle around the idea that there are three basic energies present in everything – in you, in me, in the earth and the trees. Vata, Pitta and Kapha represent combinations space and air (Vata), fire and water (pitta), and earth and water (kapha). The three energies combine in the body to create a dominant constitution and condition. Depending upon which of your own energies is dominant, various recommendations are made to help keep your particular system in balanced and harmonized. Diet, exercise and lifestyle changes might be suggested, or an herbal regimen to alter the energetic tendencies of your current system.

Contrasting with TCM, Ayurveda is considered to be a lifestyle and a system of prevention, rather than a treatment or medical system. Allopathic medicine is still recommended and considered very useful in India when the body fails to respond to the harmonizing effects of vedic therapies.

Kampo

Kampo therapy is practiced widely throughout Japan and is fully integrated into the Japanese health care system. With the introduction of Chinese texts between the 7th and 9th centuries, Japanese scholars began to adopt and fine-tune traditional Chinese herbal theories. Modern Kampo has stringent regulations and procedures that must be followed, and focuses on 148 herbal formulas that Kampo physicians find have the most profound effect on the energetic Qi system of the physical body (Chinese physicians rely on a much broader collection of formulas and texts.) Like TCM, Kampo seeks to restore balance between the five elements and the yin/yang energies so that the body can function at optimum levels. Herbal formulas are strictly regulated and overseen by the Japanese government, with very high safety and health standards.

Won-ki

Won-ki is an energetic healing system from Korea that claims to be around 5,000 years old. It combines Taoist style meditation, positive visualization, and touch therapy techniques to raise the Ki, or Qi, in the body. The idea behind Won-ki is that we are all born with a large amount of life-force in the body. As we age, this life-force is becomes increasingly drained and depleted. Unless we take conscious steps to replenish our Ki, we reach a point where it becomes fully empty, and we die.

Won-ki is taught in a simple way for very small amounts of money, making it a very positive and accessible system of healing. It is passed on to all ages: the only requirement is that one be old enough to understand and engage in speech. Proponents of the system claim that it revitalizes cells, decreases inflammation, and calms the nervous system.

Traditional Tibetan Healing

Tibetan medicine combines spiritual beliefs with traditional medical reason and logic. Herbal pharmaceutical tools are regarded as holy objects and are blessed with Buddhist prayers that invoke various healing deities. Combining Ayurvedic, Hellenic Greek, Persian and Chinese influence with two thousand years of traditional Tibetan healing methods, Tibetan medicine works with the patient's lifestyle, body, and spirit to attain healing. The primary focus is to bring the three humors, or elements, in the body into balance: wind, phlegm and bile. These humors can be disturbed by three poisons: anger, ignorance, and attachment. Spiritual dis-ease manifests in the physical body, which the Tibetan healer treats with herbs, dietary modifications, mantras, meditation and occasional acupuncture.

Scents for the Soul

Aromatherapy is the practice of using essential oils, the concentrated extracts of the protective oils and resins found in plants, to heal the emotions and combat dis-ease. Essential oils represent the first line of defense for most plants, and generally contain strong anti-bacterial and anti-fungal constituents. The best oils to use are 100% pure essential oils distilled without the use of harsh solvents.

The modern practice of aromatherapy as we know it refers both to the inhalation and direct application of essential oils. A French chemist specializing in the creation of perfumes named René-Maurice Gattefossé was the first person to coin the term "aromatherapy." In a lab accident, he became intimately acquainted with the healing powers of lavender: burned in a fragrance lab explosion, he submerged his arm in lavender oil to dull the heat. He noticed that it also subdued his pain, and his arm seemed to heal faster than ever before. This spurred him on to further investigate the medicinal properties of essential oils, and in 1928 he published a book of his findings titled "*Aromatherapie.*"

His work remained largely unknown, though it inspired a few adventurous doctors to experiment with his findings. In 1964, a French surgeon named Dr. Jean Valnet published a book on essential oils by the same name as Gattefossé, covering his own experiments using oils to treat patients with emotional problems and physically-wounded soldiers during the second World War. The world was finally ready for "*Aromatherapie*" and the field has continued to grow and gain momentum as a valid medicinal treatment since its publication, with new research every year showing that essential oils have true medicinal value.

Most essential oil properties closely mirror the healing essence of their parent plants in a concentrated form. It takes around four million jasmine flowers to create one pound of essential oil. Molecularly, essential oils are quite tiny, much smaller than cooking oils, which allows them to absorb directly into the blood stream when applied to skin or diffused and dispersed into the air. Lavender, the herb recommended for sleep pillows and nightly baby baths, yields an essential oil that is calming both for the mind and the body: lavender essential oil has been found to speed healing, lessen pain, and calm the central nervous system.

Essential oils may be used in several simple ways. They can be diffused in the air in a water-based spray or heat diffuser, or they might be dropped onto a cloth and inhaled. They are so strong that they must be diluted before using directly on the body, generally using just a few drops per tablespoon of carrier oil (such as olive or almond oil) or unscented cream base. When essential oils are inhaled, they stimulate the olfactory receptor cells and transmit the cellular information of the oil properties to the limbic system, the emotional powerhouse of the brain, which is connected to the endocrine system of the body, as well as the respiratory and circulatory systems. From there, the information is transmitted to the entire body. When applied directly to the body in carrier oil, the smaller molecules of the essential oils are absorbed through the skin and reach the bloodstream within hours, or sometimes minutes depending on the oil being used. The carrier oil remains in the outer layers of the skin, acting as an inert moisturizer.

Perhaps most significant is the fact that most, if not all, essential oils are capable of crossing the blood brain barrier. Brain tissue acts as a protective filter which most harmful substances cannot pass through. This includes the majority of medications, including chemotherapy treatments, and many bacterias. Unfortunately, this also means that dis-ease such as cancer and Lyme may not be successfully treated when it resides in the brain. However, essential oils have such small molecules that they can and do easily pass through the barrier reaching the neurons of the brain and the cerebrospinal fluid, and may be used to support treatment.

Aromatherapy has great implications for vibrational therapies. By integrating the response of the central nervous system with the entire body and mind, essential oils open the entire body to healing root causes of illness. Scientific studies have proven that smell is one of our strongest senses. Scent memories are often the strongest and most evocative, provoking sincere emotional responses. Not only do essential oils have measurable effects upon biological causes of illness, such as fungi and bacteria, but they can help our minds heal and calm our thoughts, allowing the body's natural defense system to step in and step up.

Essential Oils

Basil

Ocicum basilicum

Basil is uplifting and helps clear the mind. It is a very good herb to use when one is feeling apathetic and tired. It is associated with the heart, due to the shape of its leaves, and is believed by many people to help open the heart to love and Christ-consciousness (as characterized by unconditional love, compassion and gratitude). Physically, it may benefit liver, kidney and urinary tract problems, and is often recommended for viral and nerve disorders.

Bay

Pimenta racemosa

Long associated with manliness and strength, bay is invigorating and energizing. It is a good adjunct for cold and flu remedies.

Benzoin

Styrax benzoin

Thick and sweet with a vanilla-like odor, Benzoin has potent antiseptic properties and is a natural wound dressing. It increases circulation, also making it useful in the treatment of aches and pains. Like vanilla, benzoin has a calming, relaxing effect on the psyche, often bringing the mind back to simpler times.

Bergamot

Citrus bergamia

Bergamot is a happy, freeing scent that clears the air and cleanses space. Slightly floral and fruity, it appeals especially to children and women. Buy bergaptene-free bergamot if using the oil topically, since it may cause sun-sensitivities.

Cedarwood

Juniperus atlantica

Cedarwood is relaxing and soothing. It helps keep the psyche stable and encourages ease in everyday living. Cedarwood is considered balancing and healing for the spirit as it grounds and connects us to earth energies. Use it in oil as a soothing massage additive, or as a spray to keep away biting insects.

Chamomile, German

Matricaria chamomilla

Similar to the herb, chamomile oil has strong anti-inflammatory and anodyne properties, and will benefit muscle soreness, headaches and menstrual cramps. Apply a drop directly to swollen insect bites twice a day to reduce the pain. It is very calming to the central nervous system and often used to help induce sleep and relaxation.

Cinnamon

Cinnamomum aromaticum

Cinnamon enhances rational thought and warms the body, producing feelings of comfort. It can be used to open the soul to the abundant gifts of the universe. Do not use directly on the skin, as it can be very irritating to most people.

Clove

Syzgium aromaticum

Cloves are the calm before the storm, allowing one to bring all their energies together so that they can tackle tasks with clarity and passion. Physically, it is used to clear fungal and bacterial issues. The oil, like the herb, can also be used to combat the cystic phase of Lyme bacteria and parasites.

Coriander

Coriandrum sativum

One of my favorite oils, coriander lends clear focus and an open mind to the user. Although it sharpens the senses, it also brings one into alignment with oneself and is known to encourage easy sleep and good dreams.

Fennel

Foeniculum vulgare

Fennel oil increases energy and vitality, and balances hormones. It is believed to fortify the physical body and strengthen the auric shields. As a mild appetite suppressant, making it a perfect addition to any weight loss program. It is a mild pain reliever and anti-inflammatory, which makes it very good for healing bruises, aches and pains.

Geranium, Rose

Pelargonium graveolens

Throughout the Mediterranean you will find window boxes filled with bright geraniums. Sure, they are pretty and easy to grow, but the main reason everyone plants them? Most European houses don't have window screens, and rose geraniums help keep the mosquitoes at bay. Their scent is calming and rosy, and tends to balance male/female energies while strengthening the etheric field. Put a few drops of geranium essential oil in sprays and on pet collars to keep biting insects away in warmer months. Geranium is an amazing skin conditioner and is used by aromatherapists to treat wounds, burns, scars, bites, inflammations and infections.

Jasmine

Jasminum officinale

Jasmine is a sexy, sensual scent associated with Kama, the Hindu god of love. It allows the mind to expand and grow, to feel free. It encourages experimentation, dreaming and joyful play.

Juniper

Juniperus communis

Physically, Juniper is detoxifying and energizing. Psychically, it opens the mind to deeper states of consciousness and helps release fear-states. It is particularly strengthening for male energies and often used to clear negativity from on all levels.

Lavender

Lavandula angustifolia

As mentioned in the beginning of this chapter, lavender's anti-inflammatory and soothing properties gave birth to the science of aromatherapy. It has many applications, helping induce sleep, harmony and relaxation, as well as cleansing the emotional body. Used topically, lavender is not only a calming scent, but also a natural remedy for wounds, insect bites, rashes and burns.

Lemon Eucalyptus

Eucalyptus citriodora

Eucalyptus is widely known for its lung and sinus clearing properties, as well as it cooling nature. Lemon eucalyptus works similarly, with a stronger citrus scent that many people prefer. It

50

is a stronger anti-inflammatory and anti-bacterial agent than regular eucalyptus.

Lemongrass

Cymbopogon flexuosus

Lemongrass is a happy scent that expands the mind and encourages creativity. Use an additive to skin and house cleansers, or diffuse in the home to clear tensions and release the day's stresses.

Myrrh

Commiphora myrrha

Myrrh is very calming and evocative, opening the higher chakras and helping align us to our soul purpose. It is often used to improve the flow of Qi in the body and purify karmic residue. It is arguably one of the most blessed and world-renowned incenses: used to mummify the dead in Egypt and as a wound dressing in Ancient Greece by the Olympiads, and then given to Jesus as a babe in arms, myrrh has a grand history. Myrrh will ameliorate almost any skin problem, keep wounds closed and uninfected, and speed healing. Added to tooth pastes or powders, it is known to benefit gums and teeth, alleviating soreness and acting as an antiseptic. Myrrh tinctures can also be taken internally to help fight sore throats and minor colds.

Neroli

Citrus x aurantium

Neroli oil comes from the flowers of the bitter orange tree, and is known as one up the most relaxing and sensuous of the citrus oils. It is particularly useful when one is in crisis, suffering from loss or deeply depressed. Use it to soothe tension at the end of the work day so you can transition into a relaxed, easy, loving state.

Orange

Citrus sinensis

A perennial favorite among kids and adults alike, this makes the room smell like you've just peeled a fresh, juicy orange. It'll get your mouth watering and bring a smile to anyone's face. Bright, sunny, exuberant. These are the qualities of orange. Use it to bring happiness and warmth into your home.

Oregano

Origanum vulgare

This is perhaps one of the strongest antibacterial oils known to aromatherapists. It is used medicinally by herbalists to fight bacterial and fungal issues. As an undiluted essential oil, it can irritate skin so is best used in room sprays and diffusers. Spray in sick rooms instead of Lysol to purify the air and clean surfaces.

Patchouli

Pogostemon cablin

Patchouli is a rich, fragrant oil from a bush in the mint family. It has been prized throughout the world for centuries for its value as a base not in perfumes and a main ingredient in many incenses. It is reputed to be an aphrodisiac, and is often used to increase physical energy and vitality. It is also believed to keep away insects, particularly destructive ones such as termites and moths.

Peppermint

Mentha x piperita

Peppermint is cooling and anti-inflammatory to the body. It can be used to wake up the senses and increase mental acuity. Diffused throughout a space, it will raise the vibration and clear out old, negative energies. Purifying and invigorating, try peppermint oil to boost the body's own healing processes.

Rose

Rosa damascene

Rose oil is beloved throughout the world for its intoxicating floral scent. It has an extremely high frequency – it opens the heart chakra, calms the spirit and promotes harmony. Connecting us to our higher selves, rose vanquishes fear and sadness. This is a very healing scent to use with both the abused and those who seek dominion over others.

Rosemary

Rosemarinus officinalis

Rosemary is often used in liniments, providing heat, penetrating sore muscles and improving circulation. Rosemary works with the crown chakra and can be used to increase over-all energy, alertness, memory and even stimulate hair growth. It is often used to help remind our body of what our soul already knows: you are perfect, you are protected and all is well.

Sage

Salvia officinalis

Sage oil is both antioxidant and antiseptic, and fights fungal infections. Considered highly purifying, sage is used to clear sacred spaces and transmute negativity. It is associated with longevity and may be used to help re-awaken cells to reverse the aging process.

Sandalwood

Santalum album

Sandalwood is one of the most popular scents in the world. Its gentle, calming scent promotes feelings of safety, ecstasy and confidence. A very high vibration oil, sandalwood is believed to encourage communication with the divine, archangels and devas. Use it to align the chakras, activate kundalini and raise your vibration. Physically, it is often used to treat inflammation in the muscles and skin, as well as nerve problems.

Spikenard

Nardastachus jatamansi

Here is the oil Mary Magdalene used to anoint Jesus, mentioned in the Song of Solomon and burned in the Holy Temple of Jerusalem. A strong, heady fragrance, spikenard is used as a fixative in the fragrance industry. Known to benefit skin conditions, spikenard works on the astral plane to detoxify the aura. It has been used for thousands of years to bless and anoint those worthy of high honors, and is considered both calming and protective to the spirit. Hardy relatives of valerian, true spikenard plants are endangered at the moment from over-harvesting, so be careful where you buy your oil from, and make sure it is derived from ethically-harvested sources.

Tea Tree

Melaleuca alternifolia

A member of the large and diverse eucalyptus family, tea tree is an extremely powerful antiseptic and anti-fungal oil. Honeybees in New Zealand that feed primarily on tea trees produce Manuka honey, which has been proven to be one of the few effective remedies for MRSA, antibiotic resistant staph. Tea tree oil can be used undiluted on most people, but spot test first to make sure you are not sensitive to it. A few drops can be rubbed right on the skin onto insect bites to relieve itching and swelling, as well as applied to minor wounds to speed healing and deter infection. Its scent has an invigorating effect on the system.

Thyme

Thymus vulgaris

Thyme oil is used as an anti-inflammatory pain reliever in liniments and salves to treat sore, tired muscles. It is wonderful for respiratory conditions, opening airways and relieving congestion, and helps awaken the mind. Energetically, it is associated with both the root and throat chakras, and helps awaken the centers. It can help you forge a connection between the two, fostering grounded, clear communication and understanding.

Vetivert

Vetiveria zizanioides

One of few oils derived from roots rather than leaves, seeds or flowers, vetiver is a grounding scent that stabilizes the body and mind. Reconnect with earth energy and usher in a new era of growth and creativity with vetivert. Release your fears, be confident and deflect negativity with this harmonizing oil. Physically, use vetivert to heal tissues and help regulate hormonal activity.

Ylang-ylang

Cananga odorata

Ylang-ylang has been proven in western trials to control the production of scalp sebum, which is often a factor in slow hair growth, and even hair loss. Combine with sage for a great hair tonic, or use in scent therapy to create feelings of compassion and stimulate desire.

The Power of the Rainbow

Although the human eye can see but a small fraction of the light spectrum, we are affected immensely by the colors we see, the light that surrounds us at all time. Advertising executives and interior design consultants are well aware of this, using colors on paper and walls, in fabrics and wares, to attract us, engage us, make us laugh or bring us to tears.

Color has power: it is light, pure photon energy flowing through the universe in wave-like streams, and it resonates with every cell in our body. Multiple scientific studies have shown that these waves go through our body and are actually transformed into a useable form of energy called adenosine triphosphate, or ATP. ATP, in turn, is used by our bodies to instigate cellular repair, to process DNA and RNA, proteins, enzymes: everything our bodies need to repair themselves and exist here in the physical world. Light is, quite simply, life!

There are quite a few ways to harness light for healing. NASA uses light therapy to heal bones, benefit muscles and tissues, and relieve pain. Various forms of color therapy are believed to aid in a multitude of physical dis-eases and emotional disturbances. Personally, when I work with someone who has just suffered a painful injury, I often will place my hand on the area and imagine a cooling green light infusing it, soothing it. It's something I began doing instinctively when my first child was a toddler, getting new bumps and scrapes almost every day. I could sense most of his small bruises and injuries emitting a red glow, and found that visualizing it turning to a green light would quickly cool red glow and help diminish my son's pain. I've tried this with many people since then, adults and children, and still find it works very well. Blue light, on the other hand, seems to be better suited to chronic energetic disturbances and long-term physical issues. Every color is appropriate and helpful in the right time and place. The key is to find what works for you, and your client.

Although each chakra is generally associated with a specific color, other colors may exist or be brought into a chakra with great effect. Seeing blue, a color normally associated with the throat chakra and communication, in the root chakra may mean that the subject is very communicative and open about sexual issues, or wanting to share their personal power in a community project.

Color Therapy

Chromotherapy is the scientific term used for all applications of healing achieved through the application of color. Colors have been used as instruments of healing for over 4000 years. In Egypt, the god Thoth was believed to have first introduced this concept. Halls of healing were consciously painted to introduce the specific properties of color to intensify healing.

These days, color therapy is becoming widely accepted in modern medicine as a viable, rational form of treatment. Red light is known to benefit the treatment of wounds and cancer. Blue light is routinely used to treat jaundice in newborn infants, as well as depression and pain. In athletes, the former has been shown to amplify short bursts of energy while the latter supports sustained activity. Pink is used to subdue prisoners and measurably decrease their physical strength – perhaps we should all rethink the constant pink-ness with which we surround our daughters if we truly want them to be strong and empowered members of society.

I have one brilliant friend whose mind works a mile a minute. He has been wearing purple lenses in his sunglasses for close to 20 years now. He says he can't bear to see the world any other way. He is prone to stress and anxiety, and works in a fast-paced technical environment. These purple lenses are actually offering him an easy source daily stress reduction and emotional detox, despite the fact that he doesn't know anything about color therapy. It's no wonder he's become "addicted" to them, as he says.

To work with colors, you might choose hues which amplify or support your personality, or you might decide to use colors that balance you. If you are creative and energetic you might be drawn to green or orange – these colors will bring out your natural dynamism and creativity. If you are stressed out you might reach for blue; angry, wear more pink. If you find yourself disliking certain colors or their combinations, it could be that you are uncomfortable with or suppressing the specific energetic traits that they express or encourage.

When you add white to a color, you dampen the very aspects that it would normally encourage (hence the devitalizing effects of the color pink). When you add black to a color you lower the frequency of the color so that it is working more on a physical level than on a soul/energetic basis.

You can paint a room a specific color, use a colored light bulb or film transparency over a lamp for 15-30 minutes a day, or naturally infuse your water with color. This last method is known as hydrochromopathy, and does not involve food dyes.

All you need for hydrochromopathy is a translucent food-safe vessel for your water and sunlight. Glass is my favorite material for holding water. Choose the color glass you want to infuse your water with, fill with good drinking water and place near a window for 6-8 hours. If you do not have colored glass, a clear vessel wrapped in colored paper or plastic will work just as well. Once your water has been charged you may store it in a cool dark place (the fridge is good) and drink a glass 1-5 times a day. If you wish to preserve your color extract you can dilute it with an equal amount of 40% alcohol or 5% vinegar and store it for up to one year.

Brown

Stabilizing, grounding. It is calming and connects us to the earth and the root chakra, counteracting anger, overexcitement, and sexual addiction. Contraindications: rudeness, coarse behavior, infection.

Red

Warming, stimulating. Boosts confidence, ambition and stamina. Increases sex drive and benefits blood and menstrual issues. Contraindications: impatience, irritation, anger, wounds.

Orange

Optimistic, Energizing. Social confidence and self-assurance. Benefits respiratory issues and digestion. Contraindications: irritability, over-eating, lack of inhibitions.

Yellow

Joy. The color of the Sun combats sadness and fear. Courage, decision-making, mental stimulation, inspiration. Contraindications: ADHD, superficial interactions.

Green

Induces compassion and healing. It is a general tonic for all dis-orders. Peace, compassion, gratitude, growth (think green thumbs). Good for heart issues. Contraindications: hyper-empathy, emotional instability, inertia.

Aqua

Cooling and calming. Helps our self-expression and find our voice. Contraindications: interrupts others, talks in monologues.

Blue

Very cooling, relaxing and anti-inflammatory. Restores the basic blueprint of the physical body. Soothes ADHD. Contraindications: depression, exhaustion, insecurity.

Indigo

Very relaxing, even sleep inducing. Soothes anxiety and transports us to greater states of imagination. Benefits the eyes and ears. Contraindications: catatonia, coma, depression, spaced out.

Violet

Recalibrates the nervous system and the energy body. Induces deep sleep states, suppresses appetite and excitement. Connects to angelic healing realms. Contraindications: Boredom, depression, suppresses emotions.

Magenta/Pink

Soothing, relaxing. Relieve emotional burdens and aggression. Connect us with the power of prayer and angels. Contraindications: May dampen natural exuberance and full emotional range.

White

The full spectrum of visible light. Healing, strengthening and purifying, it is beneficial to virtually all conditions. Connects to source, spark of God-self. Contraindications: hypersensitivity, ungrounded, flighty, inactive.

Black

The absence of light, it grounds and protects us, bathing us in earth-womb energies. Use with white for significant balancing effects. Contraindications: depression, paranoia, resistance.

Ultraviolet

Antibacterial, antifungal, antiviral. Immunity boosting and healing to most systems in the body. Relieves pain and balances metabolic action. Lowers blood pressure and benefits the heart. Helps weight loss. Counteracts seasonal affective disorder and general sadness. Contraindications: skin cancer, anorexia, sunburn, vitamin D toxicity.

UV Light & Photoluminescence Therapy

Ultraviolet light waves boost the immune system and help us fight illness in the body. Although UV light can be damaging to cells in large doses (avoid sunburn, and certainly don't ever stare at the sun for any length of time!) in small, regular doses it has been shown to be quite beneficial in a variety of ways.

The fact is that we need UV light. Our bodies evolved over millennia on a planet that is bathed in sunlight every day, and our bodies adjusted to this by utilizing the sun's rays as a nutritive source of energy. 3 percent of the light given off by the sun is comprised of UV rays, which are further broken down in to UVA and UVB rays. We use these rays to make vitamin D and activate hormones, including the production of beneficial sex and skin hormones. UV light has been shown to lower blood pressure and cholesterol, and improve heart and blood flow.

Perhaps most importantly, sunlight kills germs and bacteria, and the vitamin D production it triggers in the body has been shown to be an effective treatment or preventative for many diseases, including psoriasis, tuberculosis, depression, diabetes, rheumatoid arthritis, multiple sclerosis, fibromyalgia and even certain types of cancer.

Unfortunately, at least 40% of the American population is vitamin D deficient. If you are elderly or dark-skinned, your chances double. The further north you live or the more clothing you are wear, the more time you need to spend in the sunlight you need in order to produce vitamin D and receive the healing effects of the sun. Likewise, the more pigment your skin has, the longer you need to stay in the sun. If you use sunblock, you might need to stay in the sun all day in order to process the UV rays into vitamin D. Some experts advise going in the sun for 10-20 minutes before you administer your sunscreen. Do you drink milk with added vitamin D? Don't rely on that as your sole source, unless you are drinking 8-10 glasses a day.

Photoluminescence Therapy (PT), also called **Ultraviolet Blood Irradiation (UBI)** or **Biophotonic Therapy**, was proven and taught extensively in medical schools throughout the United States until the 1950s, and is used regularly in Russia with great success to treat many ailments including viral and bacterial infections, septicemia, and even HIV/AIDS. In the US, despite over 300,000 positive clinical trials, it fell out of use during the widespread implementation of antibiotics and vaccines.

But more recently PT is finding a new scientific cheering squad, and the FDA has approved new technology from Johnson & Johnson that heralds a return to this beneficial form of light therapy. Antibiotics certainly have their place in modern medicine and have allowed much progress, but as we also discover the dangers of over-indulgence in their usage, we are also rediscovering some wonderful technologies.

So, how does photoluminescence therapy work? A small amount of blood is extracted from the patient and exposed to the UV light on the same spectrum of sunlight. This is most frequently done using a catheter and drawing the blood into a small glass chamber or *cuvette*. The blood is irradiated with UV light and then returned to the body. Most treatment methods last less than 30 minutes and treat less than 5% of the body's blood.

One of the most amazing effects of PT is that the treated blood raises blood-oxygen levels significantly. This blood is fueled with pure sun energy. It triggers cellular healing and stimulates the immune system, while creating an oxygenated environment which is prohibitive to cancer, bacteria, yeast and fungus growth. The effects of PT last can last for hours or even days; the number of treatments needed by a patient depends on the severity of their dis-ease. Many patients report an immediate feeling of improvement – generally 3-6 treatments are all that is needed to treat many chronic conditions.

The recent trials by Johnson & Johnson showed that this therapy remains remarkably effective. The company has, of course, created a machine that is much more expensive to run than previous PT setups and which is sure to make them a larger profit. But the fact remains: PT is and remains a potent medical option.

Deep Penetrating Light Therapy

Space technologies often have great applications here on earth. We've all heard about light emitting diodes, or LEDs, and how wonderful they can be for home illumination: they use far less energy than incandescent and fluorescent bulbs, contain no toxic substances (such as the mercury in CFLs), they outlast other bulb technologies by thousands of hours, and they emit almost no heat while being bright on a broad spectrum array. LEDs are perfect for use in space, because of these same factors.

People, however, don't tend to fare so well in space. Long-term space conditions cause muscles, bones and other tissues to atrophy, and injuries don't usually begin to truly heal until the person returns to earth. Is this simply low-gravity? Or is it that our bodies are intrinsically intertwined with the frequency of the earth? Regardless, a solution was needed. NASA began to look into various ways of strengthening cellular health in astronauts and other space station visitors. They had heard anecdotes about the cellular response claimed by advocates of various color ray therapies, and seen that their own plants grown in space benefitted tremendously from LED exposure. They decided to research the effects of LEDs in a variety of wavelengths on mammalian cells. And they found that people were right.

Because LEDs emit are capable of creating light on such a broad spectrum, including near-infrared light, they can benefit human cells. NASA found that the mitochondrial energy centers of cells are activated by certain colors and frequencies of light, responding positively by amping up activity to speed healing and enhance DNA replication by 150 to 200 percent. Light-emitting blanket devices can easily be used by astronauts to treat the whole body for atrophy, or small handheld devices may be used to target specific sites and injuries. Wounds, burns, bone trauma, and even cancer treatments are all the subjects of LED light therapy studies.

Studies in various hospitals in worldwide have shown that cancer patients undergoing bone marrow treatments can receive pain relief and increased healing benefits from small handheld LED devices. These small devices are now readily available for home-use, and I think they are definitely worth trying, particularly if one suffers from any sort of muscle pain or major injuries. Whether we landed on the moon or not may still be up for debate in some circles, but the efficacy of near-ultraviolet

LED light therapy for pain and tissue healing has been proven. The FDA has approved its use for "the relaxation of muscles and relief of muscle spasms; temporary relief of minor muscle and joint aches, pain and stiffness; temporary relief of minor pain and stiffness associated with arthritis; and to temporarily increase local blood circulation."

Note: There is no evidence that deep penetrating light therapy might be harmful when administered correctly. However, it is still undergoing studies as to its affect on cancers and tumors, and most experts council that direct irradiation of the eyes, thyroid, abdominal area during pregnancy, and breast tissue while nursing should be avoided until its safety in these applications has been proven.

The Iris Healing Method™

The Iris Healing Method™ is a form of light-energy healing that incorporates both hands-on and distance techniques. It combines well with all energy healing techniques, increasing healing on all levels. This method is an ancient human birthright. It comes to us through the Goddess of light, rainbows and communications, Iris.

I recently received an Iris Healing Method™ attunement through meditation with Iris, and now often incorporate this special energy into my reiki sessions, shamanic healings and vibrational remedy production process. It requires no specific training, merely the attunement which activates your ability to generate the full spectrum of light outside our normal sight range within your healing session: the light and energy of the rainbow is focused by your hands to shine directly on the subject of healing. I've found that this method gives an immense boost to regular reiki energies and augments essences with a noticeable rise in energy.

The Iris Healing Method™ uses all light frequencies, every color ray, to heal all aspects of all levels of being. It works beyond all time, in all times, healing the past, the future, and above all, now. It is pure light, Source light, pure divine energy. It connects you to Source, to the God-spark in you, to all that is good and pure in you and the universe, physical and beyond. The Iris Healing Method™ works very nicely with all forms of crystal healing and regular color therapy methods. I regularly attune students to the Iris Healing Method™ in my reiki level two and master classes.

Sound Healing

By this point in the book, we've covered most aspects of physical being-ness. Sight (color and light); Taste (foods as they relate to elemental healing and Eastern modalities); Touch (Touch therapies such as Reiki and Polarity); and Smell (aromatherapy). Hearing is the last, but by no means the least important. The sounds we create, the words we speak, carry unspeakable immutable power. Science tells us that every sound ever made exists forever, its wave-form emanating through the universe for eternity. When the bible says, "in the beginning, there was the word" this is very telling. Indeed, God is limitless, because the word will carry on forever, expanding and flowing through all time.

Brain Waves, Drumming and Change

There are four primary types of brain waves which evoke various effects at specific frequencies. These brain waves are measurable by EEG readings and are known as Beta, Alpha, Theta, Delta and Gamma waves. The brain emits all waves at all times, but is generally ruled by one type at any given moment. So while a Beta frequency may be dominant in an adult working at the computer, the other four frequencies will also be active in minute, but measurable, amounts. *As a dimensional, holographic being with many levels being, you are operating on a full spectrum of wavelengths at any given moment.*

You might be conscious of only way of being, but your soul knows better and exists in many spaces and dimensions all at once.

Beta waves are the dominant indicator of adult waking brain activity. They cycle 13-30 times per second and indicate logical thoughts, memories and sense activation. Alpha waves register at 8 to 12 cycles per second and indicate a relaxed, intuitive mindset. It is the state most commonly sought during meditation. Studies show that students perform better and develop more interest in their studies when learning from an alpha state. Theta brain waves come in at 4 to 8 cycles per second and indicate deeper trance or dream states with an active unconscious. Interestingly, theta waves also occur when we are in "fight or flight" mode, indicating a true physical autopilot in that mode. Delta waves are the slowest at 0.5 to 4 cycles per second. It is the deepest form of relaxation without dreams. Gamma waves, a fifth kind of brain activity, are the fastest at 40+ Hz. They indicate hyper-aware state of heightened perception and simultaneous thought processing. Time might seem to slow down and the subject will notice every tiny detail of his surroundings, such as often reported by victims of major accidents or traumatic experiences. People with better memories also often display more gamma waves.

In our normal waking states, humans operate at different states at different age ranges. This is significant, because as we've already shown the brain learns new behavior and gathers information more easily the slower it is cycling. Babies and toddlers brains operate almost exclusively in Delta waves. Everything is new, and everything they see, hear, touch, taste or smell becomes instantly encoded in their brain for future recall. Between the ages of four and seven years, most children are operating in Theta states. They still learn very quickly, but their

71

brains are a bit more discerning and filter out certain information if they don't want it. Primarily in the Alpha state, older children and young teenagers require an average of 21 repetitions to learn new behavior. After the age of 14 the brain waves stay primarily in the Beta range, and adults will need 1000 repetitions or more to learn new behaviors, unless they consciously put themselves into a slower brain cycle for learning. This is why affirmations, guided meditation, EFT, and hypnosis often produce such remarkable results. They repeat the message, often during lower cycle rates, over and over, until the brain finally understands that you want to encode this new behavior or idea into its patterns of belief.

Repetitive chanting and drumming are also effective techniques that still the mind and affect the brain. Scientific studies have shown that repetitive heartbeat style drumming quickly shifts brain waves to a theta range at 7hz, a deep dream state. 7hz is also the same frequency as the theta waves emanating from the earth, which means that when we drum, when we dream, we are in full vibrational alignment with the earth's living matrix. When this happens, we come into alignment with our birth purpose, with our soul's intentions and the most positive wishes of mass consciousness. This is the key to why drumming has long been used throughout the world as a tool for entering trance states, especially for healing and grounding work.

Slower brain waves have been shown to induce greater healing ability within the body, which is part of why modern medicine uses medically-induced comas to help trauma victims heal. The deep sleep-state relieves the patient somewhat from the conscious effect of pain, while a body in Delta state will experience increased Human Growth hormone, DHEA and melatonin.

Brainwave technologies exist on the market today for the purpose on engaging your brain on a specific frequency so that you can improve your daily mental state and retrain your brain circuitry. Your objective might be to become more creative, better at school, or more at peace. Choose your form of auditory brain entrainment, and get listening! Generally these technologies are not specifically recommended for pregnant women, since their potential effects on the fetus remain unknown.

Binaural beats require the use of headphones since they play a different beat to each ear. The brain registers the difference between the beats and then must mix the tones to evoke a cortical response which places the listener in the desired state. **Monaural beats** produce less stress on the brain and do not require headphones, they use two tones at once which mix before they hit the ear and are believed to produced stronger, quicker results than binaural beats. **Isochronic tones** are considered the most effective form of brain entrainment. They work by playing separate pulses of one tone through any listening device. The brain strives to synchronize with the sine waves encompassed in that tone, and thus reaches the desired wave state. All three forms of entrainment can be found online for purchase, and there are also some free videos on youtube.com. Robert Monroe's binaural beats are marketed under the name "Hemi-Sync" and benefit from decades of research at the Monroe Institute. They are also some of the most pleasant to listen to.

Repetitive **chanting** can have a similar effect to drumming and brain entrainment, inducing a meditative state and easing the transition to alpha and theta states. Tibetan monks in particular are noted for their throat-singing which allows them to emit multiple pitches or tones at once. In effect, they are some of the foremost experts in brain entrainment through the use of monaural beats.

Forks & Bowls, Not Just for Eating

Tuning forks work similarly to brain entrainment, in that they are used to produce precise sine wave patterns. Different pitches are marketed for each chakra or area of the body. Tuning forks produce very strong air impulses around them, and when they are struck near the body it is believed that the sound waves carried strong healing vibrations that travels the meridians and reaches deep tissue. Indeed, it is documented in scientific research that sound waves can and do help the body to heal, as evidenced by research on **feline purring**. Cats' purrs have been proven to heal bones and joints, increase bone strength, and relieve pain. So, if you are unwell or injured, sit with a purring cat as often as possible and allow their healing song to improve your state of being.

Singing Bowls are standing bells which are either gently struck or rubbed in a circular motion using a wooden stick. Authentic singing bowls combine several metals and are hand hammered, but these days one can find many wonderfully machine-spun bowls made from unusual metals, or even crystalline structures, which work in the same way and sound just as beautiful. They are all characterized by the ability to emit multiple frequencies at once (again performing an entrainment service). They are found worldwide and used for clearing, blessing, healing and meditating. Their sound waves emanate through the air in a tangible manner, resonating even more deeply than tuning forks and many people experience profound physical reactions to their song. Modern bowls, especially the crystal ones, may be tuned to specific chakras. In general, larger bowls have a deeper sound than the smaller ones.

Fairies, Angels and Your Inner Divine

When you begin to use vibrational remedies, you are consciously connecting to the energy that flows through everything. Vibrational remedies are, by definition, an extension of source energy, an expression of God connecting you directly to another energy frequency. By being willing to try vibrational expressions of healing, you are declaring to the rest of the Universe that you are willing to recognize ALL the energy that IS. So, at some point during your work with vibrational remedies, sooner or later, you will begin to see a bit more magic in the world. You will find it easier to sense how things are connected. Your mind will be more open to communication from your higher self, your Inner Divine.

The beauty of this is that when we receive information from our Inner Divine more clearly, miracles begin to occur. Life gets easier. The right path is more obvious. You begin to see beauty in everyone, and become less judgmental. You become more in touch with your own deeper feelings. Life flows.

The more connected you are to your own true self, the more you can follow your true life plan. You may begin to shift your routine. You might find yourself changing your consciousness in such ways that you avoid reading the news first thing in the morning so that you can stay in a better mood throughout the day. You might read more inspirational books, or spend more time with those you love and a little less time focusing on the clutter that can occur through modern living. You might find that you are less stressed, and more quiet, throughout the day. Vibrational remedies work to purify the body, allowing love to bloom and fear to fade.

Another side effect of using vibrational remedies is that you will become more open to the energies that created them. Fairies, nature spirits, devas, angels. Every being of power, grace and joy. They may begin to speak to you at night in your dreams, or simply surround you with their loving energy throughout the day. Do not be afraid to call them in to your presence when you feel you need help. They get so excited when a new human is able to sense them and welcome them into their life—you'll probably find it hard not to notice them. They are eager to co-create with us, to share their ideas and messages with us. They want nothing more than to help us help ourselves. They want only for the world to be harmonious and beautiful. They want all beings, all animals, plants, people, stones, everything on earth, to be in balance.

In order for you to easily connect with these beings, it can be helpful to understand them a little better. There is a host of information out there, but I will explain a little bit about the main groups here.

Fairies and gnomes began as regular physical entities, much like us. They were slightly higher in vibration, slightly less physical, but they were here. Eventually, they progressed to a point where they were yearning to experience a less physical existence where they could work more with the energies of life, and less with its manifestation. More with the spiritual energies of love behind the plants, and less with the flowers or trees themselves. They reside now in a vastly different plane of existence, where all is energy, and physical rules as we know them do not apply. Having been of our physical realm, they can still connect with us when it is necessary or wanted, but they can also connect more easily with Source energy.

Devas create magic with the physical manifestations of the land and the earth. They are purely non-physical beings. They play with the wind and the trees, the skies and the waters. Devas are more intimately involved in the workings of the nature of the earth. Devas have also been called nature spirits, daikinis, sprites and sylphs over the years. Each location on the planet, every little stream, each field, each flower species, every breeze has its own deva, its own spirit, complete with its own independent personality and disposition.

Overlighting angels are the angelic beings that work specifically with the Earth itself. They are in a different business than the angels with whom we are most familiar – Michael, Raphael, Gabriel, Uriel. Those guys watch over humanity. Overlighting angels watch over Gaia. The overlighting angels are more removed from than devas. They watch, and they help channel energy to the areas they watch. They speak with the devas and fairies, and feel empathy for all living creatures in their area but they do not intervene on a physical level as much as the fae. They will and do help devas and humans clear negative energy from areas when they are called in, and they do help connect humanity to Source. But they do not shift the winds or the rains or the sun or make the plants grow swifter or taller. That is the work and the play of the devas and the fairies.

Every piece of earth has an overlighting angel. Some watch small areas of earth, and some watch very large pieces of earth. Most pieces of earth have several overlighting angels watching over them, at different levels, feeling different stages of connection and inter-personal connectedness. So, as your home or street has an overlighting angel, so does your city, and the general area of your state, and the area of your country, and also your entire country. The overlighting Angels often use different boundaries than our human maps, but you get the idea. Your entire planet has an overlighting angel called the Sun, and also the Moon.

Angels and fairies can be called upon to help better connect you to the earth or other elements of nature such as the sun, moon, plants or animals. They are particularly attuned to clearing spaces, large or small. Call on overlighting angels to clear geopathic stress, or energetic disturbances in mass consciousness. Devas are great for shutting down dark streams of negative energy on your property, negative vortexes or portals to other planes and dimensions. They are wonderful for helping re-energize ley lines which have become corrupted or disturbed.

Think about the size of space you want to clean, and then call in the appropriate nature spirit(s). Always ask them respectfully for their help. They do not appreciate being ordered around, but are eager to assist us in any way they can, so long as our motives and our intent are pure. Be as clear as you can about what you would like them to do, and within minutes, days or weeks, depending on the job you set them to, you will see marked improvements. Ask if there is anything you can do in return or addition to what they are doing: sometimes you may be asked to put a specific crystal somewhere, or plant a new flower. They may ask you to take a bath in saltwater, or you may hear nothing. Often, fairies respond with a request that you clear a particular area of trash or let a small portion of your land grow wild for a particular time. Even if you do not hear the fairies or the angels speak to you, trust that they are there, and they do hear your requests. If they do not ask you for anything in return, a heartfelt "Thank you" or a small offering are always appreciated when you are finished. Joyfully, lovingly, for their hearts are pure, they seek to help humanity heal itself and heal the planet around them.

It is easy to connect to these beings, the fae, the angels. Simply call them. Put aside a few minutes in the day to relax your body and quite your mind. Breathe in deeply, calmly. Feel the serenity flow through you with each breath in, the worries and stresses of the day leaving you with each breath out. Imagine yourself on the piece of land whose angel you are wanting to contact, or holding the flower whose fairy you seek to reach. Take some time to re-create the environment you wish to be in, to really see yourself there. Now, call out (silently in your head) to the devas and fairies, the overlighting angels, whoever you wish to speak with. Perhaps you want the advice of the local fairy queen, or the spirit of your hyacinth. Perhaps you wish to speak with your cabbages and find out how to increase their resistance to insect invaders. Maybe you are seeking to speak with the Overlighting Angel of Washington D.C. so together you can work on creating a higher energy vibration in governmental spaces. Invite them in, whoever they are, and thank them for their presence and divine guidance. Tell them what it is you are seeking to know, or what you need help with. They will answer you, sometimes quickly, sometimes slowly. Be patient, and grateful for their loving, enduring guardianship of the land where you dwell.

How to Create and Use
Your Own Vibrational Essences

When you make vibrational essences you are striving to capture an energetic imprint. Most often, this is a flower, crystal or event, although you can make an essence based on practically any item or being. Want to harness the spirit of the lion? Try taking yourself to the zoo with a bottle of pure spring water and a good book, put the water as near as possible so that it can soak up the lion's energy and wait an hour or so while you read your book. Yearning to connect with the spirit of Monet? Try the same thing in a museum, or place your water on a picture of your favorite Monet painting.

Essences work on similar principals to homeopathy, and as such cannot interfere with medication or exacerbate conditions. They can only improve a situation, never harm. Flower essences can be taken by the dropperfull under the tongue or in a glass or water. They may be placed next to the bed while you sleep or in your pocket during the day. Their beneficial harmonies are far-reaching, and they do not need to be ingested to exert their influences. Try placing a few drops in the water bottle you carry throughout the day, or in your drink with dinner. Most importantly, use them with love and affection, for they will bloom under good attentions.

Flower essences are energetic infusions of flowers, made with water and preserved with alcohol, vinegar, or glycerin. The first person to bring flower essences to market was the British surgeon Dr. Edward Bach, who came up with over thirty flower essences and created a combination formula called Rescue Remedy made from five of his essences to calm the mind and ease stress on the body and psyche. He found each of his remedies within walking distance of his country home, and used them to treat his own disorders as well as those around him.

Nowadays there are many companies producing essences of many kinds: flowers, the environment, minerals, you name it. Essences are very simple to produce, and often the plants growing near you are the plants which will best heal you. Many herbalists believe that one need look no further than one's back yard for herbs: the same can hold true for flower essences. The plants I most need always seem to find their way into my yard.

Flower essences are made by filling a clean glass jar or containers with pure spring water. My favorite containers to use at home are small glass food storage bowls I bought online that came with very secure plastic lids. If I am going hiking, I like to bring small plastic bottles of spring water just in case I find a special flower.

Select the flower you wish to use, and ask the plant's permission (silently or out loud) to use it for making an essence. When you feel you have an affirmative reply, gently pluck the flower and float the flower gently on the water, or, if the flower is from a toxic plant such as Foxglove or Castor, place the flower on top of the container's lid. If you receive a negative reply from the plant, respect its wishes and move on to a different plant. Cover the container with its lid, and place in the sun for several hours. When you feel it is ready, remove the lid and the flower, and store the water in a dark glass container, mixed with vodka or brandy (any 40% or higher alcohol will generally do) in a 50/50 solution. White or apple cider vinegar may also be used. If in doubt, ask your local devas, overlighting angels, or fairies for their advice. This solution is called the "mother essence". It is what you use to make your flower essence dosage bottles. Any extra, unused essence water can be used to water your plants to great advantage.

When you wish to make dosage bottles to use the flower essence, fill the bottles with ¼ alcohol and ¾ pure water, and add 12 drops of mother essence per ounce. If you are making a combination bottle which will hold multiple essences, add 3 drops per ounce of each mother essence. Working on an energetic level, flower essences remain dormant until they are needed, so that whichever ones are relevant at the time a combination formula is taken will be activated and work for the user.

To make a crystal elixir or essence simply place the stone in a bowl of pure spring water and allow the water time to "infuse" with the stone's energies. Stones that may leach toxins should be extracted using the **indirect** method, by simply placing the stone on or near your bowl of water.

To strengthen the elixir, place it in the sun, make it during a full or new moon, a solar event or thunderstorm, or surround it with an empowering crystal grid of multiple crystal points. When you are ready, remove the crystal, and store the water in a dark glass container, mixed with vinegar, vodka or brandy in a 50/50 solution. Make your dosage bottles in the same manner that you use to make flower essences.

Environmental essences are even easier to make. All that is required is a celestial or a natural event, or a specific location.

Capture the power of the full moon by placing your bowl of water out under its light for the night. Solar eclipses, thunderstorms, hurricanes – let your water soak up their influence, and then bottle and store your essence. Perhaps you are visiting a holy site or power spot? Place your bottle of water on an altar at Notre Dame Cathedral to be imbued with centuries of powerful prayer and divinity, or by the falls of Niagara to invoke dynamic flow and cleansing. Never want to forget the happiness and inspiration you felt on vacation in Aruba? Capture the energy in your favorite spot with bottled water and preserve it with alcohol, pack it safely in your suitcase wrapped in a ziplock bag, and bring your happiness and inspiration home.

The possibilities are, quite literally, endless. You can make as many essences as you can dream of. So let's get started! In the next few chapters I will explain the healing qualities of the most commonly used flowers and crystals, as well as possible uses for environmental essences. Often you'll see things in quotes: this is information I gathered directly from the subject in meditation, the message I "heard" in my mind when I talked with a plant or crystal.

The Healing Properties of Flower Essences

Agrimony

Agrimony helps you claim your power. Are you one of those people who say yes just to please other people or avoid an argument? Agrimony can help you release your inner nervousness, the fears that you hide from the world. Helpful in combating the emotional root causes of alcoholism and drug-dependency.

Apple Blossom

"We nourish your soul. We are the star spirit, the energy of the universe. We flow through you, to you, around you. There is nothing you cannot do, nothing you need to fear. Use us when you feel alone, defeated. We will give you our power, lend you our strength. With Apple, you will be strong."

Aspen

Do you wake in the night, afraid but you don't know why? Are you nervous all the time, without any exact reason to pin it to? Aspen is a traditional Bach flower essence used to help calm your nervous system and ease your mind.

Aster

Aster stimulates and heightens communication on all levels. It can be used to increase and refine dreaming and meditation. Aster strengthens the link between the conscious, subconscious and divine selves. Truthful expression emerges effortlessly with aster, enhancing group interaction and productivity.

Astilbe

This beautiful, feathery flower heals trauma and assists with the process of letting go. It is very good to clear away patterns of addiction, victimization, and abuse. Particularly good for rescue animals.

Azalea

Joy. Love. Abundance. Azalea lifts the spirit. Turn to azalea when you are under attack, be it your body, or your mind, or your spirit. Azalea wards off foreign energies and creates a shell around your auric field. Perfect for acute viral, bacterial, or parasitic infections.

Barberry

Barberry strengthens the body, mind and soul. It takes delicate conditions and fragile energies and gives them a major boost. It raises immunity and increases our resistance -- to pain, stress, disease, seasonal allergies; anything at all that would generally weaken us loses its power in the face of barberry. Barberry works by creating an auric field of protection around the body. Tired of being afraid all the time? Tired of feeling like a victim? Feel like you need round-the-clock protection? Barberry is a great friend.

Bee-Balm, Lavender

Wild Lavender Bee-Balm relaxes the soul and allows one to let go of the stress of everyday life. It encourages "being in the moment," fostering patience and peacefulness. Great for overactive or nervous animals/people.

Beech

Beech helps you see the light and beauty of the world around you. It increases the virtues of patience and compassion, and allows you to see the good that exists in everyone.

Begonia

Begonia gently integrates the feminine and masculine together. It balances yin and yang energies in the body so that all meridians can flow properly. Because it allows energy to flow correctly, bergamot helps people become unstuck and move forward with their lives, new projects and goals.

Black-eyed Susan

Black-eyed Susan reaches into the past to create a new lineage and heal familial rifts. It clears karma and heals anger and guilt. It uplifts the dark, and transmutes it to Light. Great for animals who may suffer from genetic behavioral problems, and pack in-fighting and anger issues.

Bleeding Heart

Bleeding Heart stops the drama. It stops the pain, it stops the fear. It takes you into your heart center to see right where changes really need to be made. Do you have a hard time saying no? Hard time saying yes? This will help you either way. Stops you from making yourself a victim or a martyr and lets the truth flow straight from source to you, to the world. Let the sun shine in! Bleeding heart stops the cycles of pain and sadness, helps you release traumas and hurts, and opens up the pathways to bigger and greater love.

Bloodroot

"We are the blood of the earth mother, with her power, her energy, flowing through us. Out of our blood come purity, divinity and grace. With our blood comes healing."

Bloodroot is a potent plant with the potential to create miracles by connecting the root chakra with the heart and crown chakras. When these chakras are aligned, your other chakras benefit and flow more easily. Let your heart, your mind and your primal self come into alignment.

Bluebell

Bluebell is calming and supportive. It returns you to your center. Beloved. Simple. Peaceful. Life can be easy if you let it.

Borage

Borage heals the heart. It allows the heart chakra to expand, the energy to lift, and dark feeling of guilt or burdens to depart. It imbues one with a lightness of heart, bringing gentle light and healing to you while increasing the overall flow of source energy through your life and spirit.

Bougainvillea

Expansion. Growth. Luscious, full of life, bodacious delicious expression. Bougainvillea is one of the most creative, magical devas in the plant kingdom, ripe with vivacious energy. Tap into it, and unleash your potential.

Bull Thistle

Bull Thistle allows one to see problems and issues that are hidden and locked away deep within themselves, so that one can release and transmute them positively. Physically, it boosts the immune system.

Burr Cucumber

Burr Cucumber is joyful and uplifting. It balances the five elements in your body and allows you to release your fears and stresses by bringing them to the surface where you can see them, acknowledge them and let them go. It is a light, airy essence that brings in fairies and feelings of joyful ease.

Butterbur

"We flow with life. We help you do the same. Find comfort in your surroundings. Be comfortable in your body, in your life. Increase your self-esteem and be confident in your abilities, desires and beliefs. Allergies? Skin conditions? Headaches? These are all symptoms of your emotional discomfort and vulnerability. We help you find solace in life, so that you can be physically at ease. There is nothing on this earth that seeks to harm you. You don't need to defend your self so vigorously. Lower your guard and feel better on a day to day basis."

Buttercup

Buttercup encourages your inner child to flourish and heal. Wonderful remedy for youthful insecurities and general weakness, buttercup brings light back into the eyes and returns a sense of wonder to the user. Buttercup teaches that it does not matter what you achieve, only that you participate in the act of co-creation here on earth. It can also be used well with children who seem hyperactive or act inappropriately in public. Buttercup reassures them that they glow brightly in the world, and they don't need to act out in order to get attention.

Butterfly Bush

Butterfly bush is helpful for those approaching the end of their days; it nourishes the soul and creates feelings of bliss and fearlessness. It enhances psychic communication and mediumship and allows you to see the truth of all things.

Canna Lily

Canna is helpful for people trying to shed negative patterns, whether they stem from abuse, addiction, or anger. It revitalizes the energetic imprint of the body, helping return us to our natural blueprint. Due to this effect, it can also be used successfully to help parents better understand and keep up with their children.

Celandine

"Within us, we carry the light of the world. We can blast away tumors, heal damaged RNA and DNA, and fuel joyful expansion with our light. Take us when you are fearful, take us when you have skin issues, when you feel infected with any energy that is not yours. When

our light shines, all that is not pure and good and right flees before us. We are justice. We are pure source energy. We appear delicate, but we are strong. We are filled with the power of the sun."

Centaury

This is a good essence to combine with agrimony, as it helps you pay more attention to your own needs rather than wear yourself out trying to please others. Has your desire to help loved ones turned you into an under-appreciated house-slave? This essence will help you learn to delegate and allow others to help themselves.

Cerato

Are you unable to make your own decisions without consulting other people? Would you like to have the self-assurance to follow your own intuition? Cerato lends you the inner strength to make your own choices.

Cherry Plum

Cherry plum helps us face and transmute our dark side, allowing us to overcome irrational thoughts, fears that we will lose control and act in wild, inappropriate ways. It increases the power of light and our higher self in our physical mind.

Chestnut Bud

Chestnut Bud helps you identify karmic and life lessons the first time around, so you don't have to work through the same issue again and again. Keep choosing mates you betray you? Can't seem to keep money in your pocket when you need to? Give Chestnut Bud a try, so you can learn from your mistakes and move on.

Chestnut, Red

"Mother hen, cease your worrying. Allow others to fulfill their own purpose, as you proceed with yours. There is nothing to fear, nothing to be worrying about. Live your life, and don't worry about whether other people living as you think they should be."

Red Chestnut helps you feel joy and wonder when you watch others follow their own intuition and path, whether it is as you would choose or not. It helps you reach into your soul and feel the same pride and peace that God must feel as he watches us live and grow.

Chestnut, White

For many of us, worry is a habit. It's not an actual condition of our beliefs, but rather a condition of the mind. Our brain has been trained by movies, books, media, even school and family to focus on worry. To let the "what ifs" overshadow the here and now. White chestnut helps you release this habit and live less in fear, to turn off the gerbil wheel in your head, and experience comfort in the present moment.

Chestnut, Sweet

When the grief and the pain have become so severe that you are feeling suicidal or have completely shut down, Sweet Chestnut can help pull you back into the land of the living. Life is sweet. Let in it. Let your soul find peace right here, right now. You came to Earth for a reason. Live life. Use this essence with Star of Bethlehem for a real boost in healing grief.

Chickweed

Chickweed is a small and humble plant that nourishes the soul on a basic level by bringing in more source energy through your root chakra. It is helpful to those who have trouble sleeping through the night, fear the dark and the unknown.

Chicory

Are you the mother-hen in your office, always trying to fix everyone's problems? Do you have a hard time holding back helpful criticism, even when you know that it isn't wanted? Do you try to keep everyone you love as close as possible, fearful of losing the connection should they move too far away or become too independent? Chicory will let you allow others to live their life freely and joyfully, with you by their side as a co-creator rather than as the director or caretaker.

Clematis

Clematis flower essence fights tumors and growths in the body, and distortions of the mind. Ill thoughts, depression, and corruption all benefit from Clematis. Clematis opens the higher chakras in short bursts, re-aligning them with their soul-purpose as they are cleansed. The mental and etheric bodies also benefit from Clematis, allowing miasms and karmic and genetic distortions to be re-programmed and wiped clean.

Clover

Clover essence aids digestive disorders stemming from a lack of self-love or acceptance. It heals familial rifts and feelings of resentment, particularly against the mother. Clover may also be used to help access and encourage one's feminine, nurturing side.

Columbine

Connect to the spirit of the green man, the dwarves and the fairies with Columbine, which is most beloved by the earth elementals. Columbine lifts the spirit and mends fragile, egos. It is particularly well suited for insecure teenagers. Physically, it strengthens fragile bones, connective tissues and the circulatory system while it mends the psyche.

Coreopsis

Coreopsis is Joy and Laughter, and alleviates stress and worry. It also works with the digestive and urinary systems, and is very good for nerve or stress disorders.

Crab Apple

Crab Apple helps clear miasms, dis-ease, and toxins from the physical body, while helping the mind and spirit identify issues that need to be released. This remedy helps you release those issues with grace and ease, and focus on reality with clarity and peace.

Crocus

"We are the first. The bravest. The most daring. We take all the energy that has been stored in the earth and use it to burst out of the darkness of winter before all others, to bloom brightest when no one else will dare. Work with us to grow stronger and braver, to face adversity head on with fearless resolution."

Dahlia

Do you want to connect with the Greek and Roman gods, the old ones? Dahlia is for you, as it connects us to our earthy, powerful selves. Dahlia bolsters both the root and crown chakras, allowing us to act with true purpose. Dahlia also helps open the Akashic records to us in the dreamtime, increasing our powers of both and inner and physical sight.

Daffodil

Daffodil creates a protective shield around the body. Feeling uneasy, worried or distressed? Try Daffodil. It is both reassuring and expansive, creating a brighter outlook in life along with feelings of safety and security. Physically, daffodil benefits digestive disorders and reflux. It optimizes the assimilation of both nutrients and ideas.

Daisy, Gerbera

Antisocial? Feeling like a wallflower? Wishing you could get noticed or just shine a little brighter? Gerbera Daisy helps you stand up and stand out. People you haven't spoken to in years may come out of the woodwork, clamoring for your time and attention. The boys at the club will wonder, "What is it about her?" Gerbera daisy brings out your natural light and beauty, and helps foster truer, deeper connections with other people.

Daisy, White Shasta

White Shasta Daisy brings out the wild, childlike joy in you. It creates good bonds with children, for then you can see how they see. It restores innocence and purity. Helpful for childhood illnesses and traumas, as well as for aging.

Daylily

Daylily reminds you to delight in everyday, ordinary moments. It heals reproductive organs and traumas, and also re-creates familial bonds in a more positive way.

Dogwood

Dogwood carries the strength of purity. With dogwood, you can be reborn, rebirthed. Dogwood detoxes and removes impurities from the system. It sings of beauty and perfection, it lures your cells into the wonder of creation; it returns your body to youthful vibrancy and a state of true renewal. It allows your soul to shine through with pure, undiluted radiance.

Echinacea

"Echinacea harnesses the power of the pyramids, the light of the divine, and the magic of the ancients. We are the harbingers of growth and progression. You know that we improve health when we are taken as an herb. This is because we literally amplify the energy signature of the soul within the body, and move the body closer to the perfection that humanity is moving ever-towards. You are looking to ascend, to perfect yourself here on earth? Work with our essence. We are the beginning of the best path you can take."

Elder Flower

Elder Flower connects you to the fairies and nature devas. The best time to make this special essence is on the Summer

Solstice, the longest day of the year and a time traditionally linked with fairy revels. Legend has it that if you rub elder flower water on your eyes at the solstice, you will gain "fairy sight" or the ability to see the fae. In particular, summer solstice elder essence links you to the full power and dynamism of the sun, and is helpful to all those seeking to study herbalism, the druid arts, or other mystical schools of knowledge. Elder flower stimulates energy, vigor, resilience, joy, and our powers of renewal. A very good essence for animals and people who are recovering from a prolonged illness, elder is also helpful for those who are "feeling their age" or looking to feel younger.

Elm

Are you feeling overwhelmed by life? Overburdened or not quite up to the task you have set for yourself? Elm is an angelic, supportive essence that benefits all those who wish to do good deeds and benefit humanity or the world in some way.

Evening Primrose

Evening Primrose balances the male and female aspects of the self, and also fosters easier relationships between the sexes. It encourages openness and honesty, truth and trust. Good for those who have a hard time entering relationships, as well as animals involved in breeding or mixed-sex packs. Evening primrose helps create a strong, dependable foundation to support the lightness of beauty of joy with ease.

Fern

Ferns have been here since the beginning of time. Larger, towering ferns created forests on earth and fed dinosaurs of all immense proportions. Let fern return you to the power of humanity. Be re-born with full possession of the divine blueprint of man and unlock your true potential. Right now, we use 10% of our brains. We used to use more. Would you like to see what you can do? Let fern begin your initiation.

Flowering Raspberry

Flowering Raspberry is an interesting wildflower. Its huge, dew-dropped leaves are reminiscent of sycamore foliage, and its tart raspberry-colored fruits can be used to make a drink like pink lemonade. An essence made from its large magenta flowers will draw the sweetness of life to oneself. It revitalizes the mind and clears "fuzzy" thinking. Benefits aging animals and people.

Foxglove

Foxglove is for healing any trauma in the past future or present. It heals all wounds on all levels. It opens the heart for healing and shields from negativity. It lends strong, supple resilience to those who take it.

Gaillardia Aristata

"Who are we of the gaillardia clan? We are the small yet hearty, the rugged beauty of the American wastelands and deserts brought into your

garden to spread laughter and amusement. We bring you strength, courage, fearlessness. We help those in times of need, in times of trouble, to find their center. We ground you, increasing energy and stamina, while cleansing your aura with light. Behold us, and laugh! Behold us and be at ease!"

Gentian

Gentian strengthens the stomach chakra, bringing self-confidence and determination to those who need it. Good for digestive disorders, and to help calm nervous feelings which manifest in the abdomen.

Gladiolus

Gladiolus activates the kundalini and fires the soul, raising the vibration of the body simultaneously. It clears mass consciousness, facilitates transition and enables ascension. Helpful for auto-immune diseases and fatigue.

Gorse

Gorse, as those who have worked with the energies of the Findhorn Sanctuary in Scotland know, is an extremely rugged, strengthening flower energy. It survives in the most barren, hopeless conditions to bring beauty to the earth and fire up the soul. Use gorse when you've lost all hope, when you feel nothing can be done, when you are ready to give up. Gorse would never, never give up. Gorse will lift you up and make you strong.

Heather

Do stay in relationships merely for the sake of company? Are you afraid to be alone? Heather helps you appreciate yourself and your own company. It will bolster your self-confidence and help you find joy in quiet, intimate moments alone with your own thoughts. You are free. You are wild. You are a joy to look upon, a unique beauty borne of spirit and light. Reach for the joy you are due. Never settle for less.

Holly

Holly essence empowers and balances the five elements within you to create strong clearing effects. Parasites, miasms, dark beings and genetic disturbances scurry and flee before it. Damaged cells are purged and you are left feeling clean and clear. Traditionally, holly essence is used to heal and expand the heart chakra, and to alleviate anger, rage and envy while generating acceptance.

Hollyhock

Hollyhock clears and connects all chakras in all the bodies: etheric, astral, physical, spiritual, mental. It allows one's life path to blossom and unfold as it was intended. It is very healing to all physical issues, including chronic disease and allergies.

Honeysuckle, Flowering Vine

Honeysuckle works on the physical to heal cancers and immune disorders. It repairs RNA and DNA and helps transition the body into a LIGHT-body, a crystalline form. It allows you to embrace the present and look forward to the future, releasing any beliefs that the best part of your life might be over or that you cannot achieve your dreams.

Honeysuckle, Northern Bush

Northern Bush Honeysuckle heals RNA and DNA just as all honeysuckle do, while realigning mass consciousness with the earth and all new, higher energies on this physical plane of existence. It allows for full ascension progression and pulls in the help and healing powers of all the angels and nature devas.

Hornbeam, or Ironwood

Hornbeam is strong. It is regal. There is nothing you cannot handle. You are all you need. You are irrepressible, completely sufficient, and fully worthy of all your dreams. Hornbeam can help you feel it, see it, be it.

Hosta

Hosta brings deep wisdom from the divine. It connects you to higher sources of knowledge, and accesses many "records" including the Akashic and Atlantean. Brings aged wisdom to animals or people who act a bit "goofy" or "spacey."

Hummingbird Vine, aka Trumpet Vine

Hummingbird vine allows the crown chakra to interact fully with the root and sacral chakras. This results in improved self-expression and higher clarity in personal relationships and sexual situations. Hummingbird vine gives you the courage to say what if on your mind, and the confidence to deliver your ideas effectively and with eloquence.

Hyacinth

Life is sweet. It is a process, and hyacinth is here to help you accept all aspects of this process. Birth, life, death. Hyacinth helps you see the sweetness in all situations. It allows you to get past the drama, past the pain or frustration, and find the greater lesson in your current experience. You will see the lesson, and move past it, into the light and the beauty of your next experience, your next lesson.

Hydrangea, Indigo/Violet

"Speak to us. Give us your worries, your fears. Let us transmute them. Let us soothe you. You simply need to reconnect to your highest good, your highest self, your most natural and beneficial state of being. Let us repaint your aura with the vibrant tones of light that are most natural to you. Let us help you reconnect with your spiritual birthright. Insecure? We can help. Bullied? Fearful? Shy? We are here for you."

Hydrangea, Pink

"We all, the hydrangeas, lighten the heart. We are all loving, giving energies that re-light the aura and re-ignite soul connections. When we are pink, as I am, we tend to direct more of our love and healing to your heart center, as opposed to our blue and violet friends who focus more on the state of your mind. We look after matters of the heart. Let us heal you. Let us connect you to love, to pure source energy, that which so many of you call Christ Consciousness. We are here for you."

Hyssop

Hyssop has been used since ancient times to purify the body and soul. Use it to release old feelings of pain, anger or guilt. It cleanses DNA and allows your third eye to access and clear old karma. Physically, Hyssop also purifies the body, and helps fight bacterial and viral infections. Spray it around the home to create a better, lighter atmosphere.

Impatiens

Rush, rush, rush. This is the remedy for the 21st century. We want everything done right away, on our desk "yesterday", messages replied to instantly. Many of us are impatient, suffering road rage, too hungry to wait 20 minutes for a home-cooked meal, too busy to spend quality time with those we love. This remedy helps you live a bit more slowly and easily, without the rushing or impatience. It has a long tradition of benefitting those who have a hard time waiting for others to finish a task, preferring to work on their own and do it themselves rather than watch the "inefficiency" of others.

Iris

"We are the doorway to the other realms, the way to the heavens and dimensions unseen. Use us to get to the other side of the rainbow. Reach new heights of perception, and see beyond the veil to reality as it could be, as you want it to be."

Iris allows you to reach into yourself and harness all your creative powers, to see truth in all matters and release blockages that have been holding you back.

Jewelweed

Jewelweed releases guilt and blame. It travels with Poison Ivy for this very reason: for poison ivy grows to remind us of the dangers of violence against other living beings, jewelweed is here to help us alleviate any deep-seated guilt or anger we may feel from violent events, whether from this lifetime or another. Expect great shifts in consciousness when you use this remedy!

Lady's Mantle

Use Lady's Mantle Flower Essence when you have difficulty calming your sympathetic nervous system, whether from shock, electrical interference or emotional trauma. The Lady helps when you are feeling anxious, hyperactive, or have high blood pressure, calming the heart and spirit. She softens protection around the physical heart to allow healing energy into your heart chakra and emotional body. She helps regulate the female sexual organs and offers nurturing compassion to all so that we may align with our higher selves. Lady's mantle also helps regulate the action of water in and upon our physical body.

Larch

Afraid of success? Feel like a failure? Larch bolsters self-confidence and helps foster the drive you need to move forward and achieve your dreams.

Lilac

Lilac is a soothing flower remedy – good to help you sleep, good to calm airways and nervous reactions. Lilac is also helpful when you are trying to reclaim lost memories, be they from this lifetime or the last. It is uplifting and relaxing, helping to draw good things to you. Physically, lilac can be used to release soreness from the back, especially to soothe tight shoulders and necks.

Lupine

Lupine is wild, unfettered, unrestrained. It brings out your primal power and strength. It calms flight or fight responses and allows you to face life with ease and an open heart.

Magnolia

Magnolia brings together male and female archetypes, in particular the emperor and empress, the mother and the father. Magnolia is regal, enduring. Use magnolia when you need to be heard, when you want to be taken more seriously. It lends an aura of authority and assurance to those who work with it, and helps you to work with the system, rather than against it, to achieve your heart's desire.

Maple

"Sweet, strong, loving shade. When you cut us, we give you our love. Use us to make you strong, yet supple. You can be in charge, yet be kind and sweet, too."

This is a wonderful remedy for parents who feel overworked or burnt out.

Milkweed

Milkweed opens your heart chakra and reactivates the thymus gland. It gives you the courage to blossom and let your true colors shine forth. Face your true self with confidence and release addictive behaviors.

Mimulus

Release your fears. This is a wonderful remedy for small children and animals suffering from night-terrors, separation anxiety or fearing thunderstorms. Fears of loss, pain, darkness – all benefit from the small, yet strong, mimulus. Mimulus sheilds people who feel defenseless.

Mountain Laurel

Mountain Laurel blocks geopathic stress and encourages resilience. It is the essence to use during epidemics and disasters to heal the heart and strengthen the psychic shield. It brings in the protection of the angels. Anytime one is in a new situation and needs a little boost of confidence, this is a good essence to use. Wonderful for children or animals suffering from separation anxiety or feeling bullied others.

Mullein

Mullein opens one to channeling and facilitates better communication with one's greater self and the Divine. It clears away mental debris and silences inner chatter so that one can "hear" the big picture. Healing for ear problems.

Mustard

This is the remedy to reach for when you are in your deepest despair, your darkest hour. When you can't bring a smile to your face, when all efforts at happiness leave you feeling empty, mustard has the ability to bring the power of the sun into your soul. It is bright, it is happy, it is healing.

Oak

Oak is a perfect ally for those who are already strong, already fighting a good fight, but needing a little more help in their corner. The spirit of the oak is strong, inviolable, unfaltering. It helps you keep your fire stoked, your love strong, your will unbending. With oak, your aim is always true.

Olive

You know how the cultures of the Mediterranean are so well-known for their joie de vivre? It's no coincidence that their diet has been high in olive derivatives for generations. They have, over years and years, literally harnessed the power of olive to enliven their DNA and create cultures where life revolves around joy, and daily work goes hand in hand with pleasure. This is the power of olive, the power to show you that physical life is not the enemy of your soul. Physical reality is an opportunity. It is life. It is a gift. Enjoy it!

Partridge Pea

It is possible to be sensitive and strong, open and protected at the same time. This is an essence that widens the corridors of communication between Nature and Man, devas and reason. Trying to see fairies or plan a new garden in harmony with nature? Looking to become more at peace with the Earth? Partridge Pea is the essence for you.

Pine

"Pine endures. It keeps its needles throughout all odds, throughout all seasons. It never fails, it never fades. It is a gift of the forest, a gift to the world. **So are you.** *No matter what you think you've done, no matter how you feel you've failed, you have not. You are perfect, just as you are. Move on. Continue to live. Endure. You will always be pure, perfect spirit, and you are the power and the glory of God."*

Peony

Peony lightens the load. Take your heavy burdens and let them go. Peony shows you that it won't do you any good to stay tied down to your worries and fears, and helps you shift your focus to possibilities and goals.

Petunia

"We, the Petunias, are a most energy among the plants. We hold incredible vitality. We are fire and water blended most harmoniously. We are here to boost your ability to perform when you feel constrained, to do everything you are wanting no matter the odds. Do you feel like your life, your work, your situation "stinks"? Use us to work within the establishment, shift your reality, allow the world to see and rejoice in your full vitality and power. Use us and see how wonderful life can be with just a few small, simple shifts. Be FULL-filled. Be blessed."

Poppy

Poppy works with the mind to heal old traumas, and help you overcome chronic conditions that cause pain and discomfort. Use poppy to ease the mind and body and sleep more easily. It is useful for those going through the grief process.

Rhododendron

Use this flower to help cure shyness and insecurity. Rhododendron boosts self-confidence and allows you to accept yourself independent of how others think of you. You are beautiful and perfect just as you are. Rhododendron helps you see that, feel that. Helps you *know* it in your bones.

Rose, Climbing

Climbing Roses are for manifestation and creation. They help with the ascension process and to bring abundance on all levels into one's life. This rose reaches into the future to manifest your desires quickly and potently. Heals by blessing one with the Holy Spirit.

Rose, Joseph's Coat Climbing

Joseph's Coat Climbing Rose connects you with the divine, and allows you shift your consciousness more easily. It aids in transitions of all kinds, and helps you allow miracles into your life. It is a major energizer physically, facilitating the healing process.

Rose, Miniature

Miniature Roses help you see the big picture. They bring a love of all things to your heart, and expand your heart chakra. They are pure love, bringing love to those in need.

Rose, Rock

Rock rose is for use in acute, extreme situations where you fear for the safety or health of yourself or another. You can even use it on the unconscious or delirious by placing a bit on the lips, cheeks or the forehead. It helps us return to our perfect state of soul-ness, whether that is to be here, now, in the physical, or if we are passing on and need help easing our transition.

Rose of Sharon

Rose of Sharon connects you to Christ energy. The joy contained in this flower is ever blossoming, never fading. It lifts you up in times of sadness and reminds you of the Oneness of all things. Clears guilt and anger, restores purity of heart. Good for both the abused and the abuser.

Rose, Wild

Wild rose returns you to your original, energized soul state. Remember what you felt like when you were a child, a teenager? Nothing could hold you down. You were free, unfettered, and you knew it. You may not have known exactly where you were headed in life, but you knew that it was supposed to involve joy and excitement. Life is not about giving up your dreams. Life is not about settling for second best. Life is, quite simply, for living. Go for it! Let wild rose take you by the hand and lead you there.

Scleranthus

Wishy-washy? Unable to choose between one or the other? Stop going back and forth between decisions, lovers, jobs, whatever. Scleranthus helps you make up your mind with clarity and decisiveness. It gives you strength to follow the path with a heart, to dream the impossible dream. Go forward, fearless one, and doubt not what you have chosen.

Siberian Squill

Be easy. Be calm. Release your anger. Siberian Squill helps you transmute anger into joy. It releases emotional hang-ups that have been stored in your body and are affecting your liver, spleen and pancreas. It helps you communicate and let go of the pain and resentment. Squill sets you free from your inhibitions and self-impose obstacles, so that you can move forward with a sense of joy and freedom.

Squash Blossom

Squash Blossom frees you. It expands your creative potential by raising your vibration and pumping up your aura, large, larger, largest. It gives you the strength to be yourself. Wonderfully healing for the shy and scared.

Star of Bethlehem

Star of Bethlehem brings comfort to those in need. This is the remedy most often used for those going through the process of grief and loss. When you can't move on, when you can't go on, this is the remedy that can help you process your emotions. Find relief. Feel joy. It is possible to feel it again.

Sunflower

Sunflower is huge, yet humble. Its only real desire is to help feed your soul. It transmutes the darkness into light, night into day. Fear becomes ease, depression becomes happiness. Sunflower is beneficial to all, uplifting and nourishing to all layers of the body: physical, astral, energetic, mental, spiritual.

Tamarack

Tamarack will toughen you up. It helps to strengthen the whole body and tone your mental faculties so you can do what you need to do. It helps you align with the new earth energies and balance the any excess kinetic energy in the physical body. Use it to combat geopathic stress and target a weak spleen or liver, or to help boost confidence and overall stamina.

Tiger Lily

Tiger Lily shows that there is wisdom in folly, strength in laughter, truth in joy. It helps one let go of disapproval and feelings of inadequacy, and reminds us that we are all unique and necessary in the grand design, the Divine Tapestry of Life. Also good for digestive issues, and alpha animals that are too tough or dominant.

Tomato

"The fruit which we bear nourishes you, so many of you, but so few take the time to notice or appreciate our little flowers. Thank you. Thank you! We are happiness, we are clarity. We would share it with you. The health of our fruits is debated and praised by many, but what you need to see is that they are healthful only when you appreciate the entire plant, the entire process that created us. So it is with all plants that create food. If you see only the result, and do not appreciate the entire energy of the plant, you are missing so much! So we have come to you as a flower essence to help you connect to this process, to the energies of tomatoes especially, but also ALL food plants, so that you may better assimilate nutrients and benefit your health with ever bite you eat. Our essence will make you more naturally appreciative and blessing of all your food. So be it."

Tulip

Tulip connects us to our inner-child. It is protective and loving, and allows us to greet life with child-like wonder and innocence once again. Life is not all about perfection. Tulip reminds you how to play. A wonderful remedy to support all children and animals, and those who work with them.

Vervain

You think you are confident and strong-willed. Others sometimes use the words stubborn and rigid. If you are looking to loosen up a little and broaden your mind, give Vervain a try. It will help you learn how to think outside the box, to see the broader picture.

Vine

Persistence. Tenacity. Drive. These are the watchwords of Vine. Vine engenders success and energizes those who take it. Beneficial to use during long-term, weakening illnesses or when undertaking daunting projects.

Walnut

So. You have a dream. You know what you want and how to get it. But you're slightly doubtful because you hear or fear what other people think and say. Walnut toughens up your defenses. It weaves a beautiful shell around you that will strengthen both your aura and your mind. You can be and do whatever you want. You cannot be broken, you cannot be bound. Reach for the stars, filled with sweetness, love and joy. So what if some people think you're a little nuts?

Water Violet

Water Violet brings peace and quiet to those who need it. Soothe your babies. Ease your mind. Be calm. Be free from the noise and drama of the world.

Weeping Wiegela

Weeping Wiegela is a special flower that allows you to try again and succeed. It shows you that it is never too late to bloom, and that karma and genetic lineages can be cleared and as if they never existed. You are the creator of your reality, anything is possible. Benefits genetic and "incurable" diseases, also depression.

Wild Oat

Looking for success, but unsure where to begin? Wild oat takes pure, undirected energy and helps you find direction.

Willow

Don't be bitter. Be brave. You don't need to be angry at life, God, or yourself. You can have a second chance at happiness, but you need to let go a little first, and allow yourself to heal. Willow helps soothe the pain so that you can begin to heal. Wonderful for trauma victims, widows, anyone who has lost or been hurt in any way. Willow puts you on the road to healing, soothing the aura and rebuilding trust in the universe.

Wood-Sorrel

Wood-Sorrel clears debris from your past and your present path so that you can see you way clearly. It returns you to a state of child-like perfection and anticipation. Particularly good for abuse and neglect victims, so that they can become happy, self-empowered fulfilled individuals.

Yarrow

Yarrow is extremely strengthening. It helps heal energy leaks in the body. If someone is draining your energy, yarrow makes it impossible for them to continue tapping in to you. When you are suffering from bio-energetic or geomagnetic disturbances, yarrow helps you adjust your frequency so that you feel comfortable and stable. Great for those working in stressful situations or on the computer all day. Also helpful for blood and circulation issues in the body.

Yucca, Adam's Needle

Yucca Filamentosa, or Adam's Needle, is a perennial hardy yucca that grows wild and joyfully free. Yucca encourages you to reach for your inner heights of being, to easily become the best that you can be, spiritually and emotionally. Yucca will help you dispel anger and stress by illuminating your safety of being at its very core. Nothing can harm you. You are invulnerable, safe, and inviolable.

Zinnia

"Be bold. Be bright. Go forward and shine! You came here to live, to love, to laugh and just be. So do it. Be it! Let us play with you, and be with you. We will give you power and courage, the ability to abandon yourself to your true self. To walk your path with confidence and without fear or doubt. We will lift you up and help you be who you are."

How to Work with Crystals

Minerals have been used by healers for thousands of years, perhaps for as long as man has been interested in tools. Crystals and rocks carry the soothing, grounding energy of the Earth within them. Each stone has a different crystalline structure which resonates at a unique frequency, and each frequency targets a different healing energy. Some crystals are used for healing, some for calming, some for joy and some for protection. Many great books exist about crystals: my favorites are "The Crystal Bible 1 & 2" by Judy Hall and "Love is in the Earth" by Melody. The first are beautifully illustrated references with all the most common stones, well-suited for beginners and collectors alike, and the second is a vast compendium of practically every stone ever named.

Collecting crystals can be an addictive pastime; their energies are so uplifting and expansive, generally altering our vibration in many positive ways. When you are looking for new stones, whether it be on a walk in the woods or in a metaphysical store or at a jewelry expo, let your senses guide you. Listen to your inner mind and pay attention to any small tugs you may feel. Not only can we feel crystals, but they can feel us. The right stones will recognize your energy and call to you.

Many people like to clear or purify their new stones of previous handler's energies. This can be done by placing the stone in a bowl of cool water (you may add a little salt, which is very purifying) or letting the light of the sun or moon shine on it for a prescribed amount of time, be it hours or days. Sunlight or strong fluorescent light can fade the colors of some crystals, such as amethyst and fluorite, so use care.

Before working with your new stone, quiet your mind. Sit with your stone in your hand and allow yourself to feel its energies. You can program your crystal by conversing with it and asking it to help you achieve a certain goal, chanting your intentions over it, or stroking the stone while you state your purpose. Place the stone on a piece of paper on which you've written a prayer or goal, or put it in your pocket or on your alter or under your pillow, and allow it time to work its own special creation magic.

Supporting stones can also be placed near your sleeping area, in or near your drinking water (use care, as some stones can be toxic or deteriorate in water, such as malachite, sulphur and selenite), worn around your neck or carried in your pocket. They can be used when you are conducting hands-on healing work, or placed near your tinctures and remedies for extra empowerment. Used in the environment, crystals may heal harmonic discord and can even ameliorate EMF waves. They are soothing and beneficial to all beings, on many levels.

Grounding with Crystals

Stones, used properly, are an obvious and powerful choice for grounding your energy. Of the earth, they are good channels for free-floating energy. The key is to pick the right stone for your purpose. A meteorite, such as moldavite, may be beautiful and intriguing, but it is not going to bring you back down to earth. Pyramid shaped stones, like naturally-occurring apophyllite or carved pyramids, raise energy and open the crown chakra to the heavens, but do nothing to connect that heavenly energy to the body's lower extremities and down through the earth.

Most stones used for healing by the new age community in general are not grounding. They do wondrous and beautiful miracles. They connect us with the higher planes. They bring love and healing into our lives. Many of them do clear the chakras and the body, but few are adept at helping to ground us. By using only stones that open us, and not combining them with grounding, protective stones, we are left open to mixed messages and misdirected energy.

I recommend that everyone who works with stones always have a few good grounding stones on hand: carnelian, obsidian, hematite, tiger's eye, smoky quartz, onyx, agate and jet are some good choices to begin with.

Gridwork with Crystals

A crystal grid is a number of crystals arranged into a particular geometric form creating a particular energy field. The simplest crystal grid is a triangle formed of three crystals. When you form a crystal grid, the crystals should be of equal strength and similar size. You can form a grid of any geometric shape or symbol. Each shape and symbol carries its own symbolism and uses. You may use a grid to charge or empower any object, including another crystal or yourself, by placing the object in the center of the grid. Try focusing your intent by choosing tarot or oracle cards, or writing a list of desires, and placing them within the center of the grid.

Crystal grids enhance the power of your intention. They are far more powerful than any one single crystal, as the energy of a group always adds up to more than the simple sum of its members. Use grids to send energy to others for long-distance healing, to broadcast your desires to the Universe or to increase the charging power of your essences. Grids can be used to create strong protective boundaries or to clear and charge simple items like your food. Place crystals in particular spots around your home to create a beneficial living grid.

The simplest grids are crystals placed in a circle around an object at regular intervals. But the possibilities are only limited by your knowledge of geometry and sacred designs. You can use shapes like the triangle or star, or more complicated forms based on holy objects like the Ankh of the Flower of life. For a prosperity spell you might use a plus sign or a dollar sign. For healing you might employ a simple circle or use the caduceus, the medical symbol of Asclepius's staff with a snake winding around it. You may choose to use a picture of the person you are healing with the essence in the middle and the stones placed on important chakra or meridian points in the image. Some people like to draw their grid on paper first, or use string or wire to lay out larger diagrams.

The important thing to remember is that you are creating a framework for the power of the stones to communicate with each other and to harness their full potential. You might leave your grid up for an hour or for months. Continue to work and pray over the grid until you feel its work is done. Only you can know how long this must take. You might time your gridwork to coincide with a powerful solar eclipse or a full moon, or you might use seven days to heal seven chakras.

By aligning the crystals into a geometric form, they form beams or vortices of light and energy within the center: it is with this energy field that you are working. Eventually you may want to build crystal grids under your bed or chair, or on a specific part of your body that may be ailing you: wait until you feel ready to process the energy generated by crystals to try this. If you feel you have taken in too much energy afterward, try holding a grounding crystal such as agate, carnelian or obsidian; take a salt bath; or take a walk in nature.

Crystal grids can absorb imbalanced energies and are excellent tools for healing but as always you should clear the crystals using sun or moonlight, running water, salt water, smudge or earth. Always ask their permission before you conduct this sort of work. And enjoy yourself!

A Meditation for Accessing a Crystal's Spirit

To begin, sit comfortably and hold your stone in your hands, taking three deep breaths.

Breathe in, and breathe out.

Relax your muscles.

Breathe in and out.

In and out.

Calm your mind, release your thoughts.

Allow your entire being to relax.

Easy. Easy.

Calm.

Feel your consciousness sinking, safe and slow, as you go deeper and deeper into the darkness of your inner mind, as you reach your inner point of stillness.

Here in the center of your being, deep in your mind's eye, see yourself quiet, at peace, and whole. See yourself stand up, and walk through the darkness into a cool cave deep in the earth.

You feel safe here, secure, and very protected.

You run your hand along the walls of the cavern and can feel the vast wisdom of the ages surrounding you.

In the middle of the cave, you see the great mother of the stone you are holding, the piece from which your own was birthed, and you approach it with reverence.

It welcomes you to the cavern, and asks you to sit and speak with it.

You show the mother stone the small piece you hold in your hand, and ask her to bless it.

Ask the stones if there is a particular name your piece would like to be addressed by, and introduce yourself. Explain what your intentions are, and what you are currently desiring in your life or needing help.

Ask the stones what way would be best for you to work with your piece, and if it has any particular messages for you.

Thank the mother and your stone for their blessings and their help.

Stand up, and walk back the way you came. See yourself deep in the darkness, deep in your body, once again.

Breathe deeply.

In.

And out.

In and out.

Relax.

Return.

The Healing Properties of Crystals

Agate

All agates are gently grounding, and soothe and calm the nerves. They help build confidence and self-reliance. Agate comes in almost every color, each of which corresponds to different chakras to further help with chakra specific issues. For example, green agate is known to be especially healing, very beneficial for the heart and lungs, and while helps connect you to live plant energy. Red agate is grounding, while yellow agate clears the aura with sun energy. Agates are particularly well-suited for children and pets, due to their gentle, nurturing disposition.

Alexandrite

"We are a stone of JOY. We are the stone to bring you into alignment with your true self. We are the stone that helps you be at one with your higher self, to be at one with all of you, and all of us. For this reason, we have received a reputation as a channeler's stone. It is because we hold pure source energy. Pure Source YOU."

Alexandrite fosters intuition and creativity. It helps us move past moments of sadness and hopelessness, and can be very helpful when trying manifest your dreams. On a physical level it stimulates the pineal and pituitary glands, and benefits brain function.

Amethyst

Amethyst is probably one of the best-known crystals in the new-age community. It helps open the third eye and enhances psychic awareness. Physically, it also benefits the entire head and brain, making it useful for migraines, hearing issues, and nerve disorders. It is a great stone to help tune you in to your higher self and trigger cellular renewal and evolution.

Apatite

"People mistake the stillness of water for calm, but we are not calm. We are deep. We hold the mysteries. We hold the energies of the unfathomable and the potentials of the void. Blue is the color of life force. It is the color of that which animates and holds together all life energy on your planet, all that is alive in the universe, all that thinks, feels, moves, grows and glows. We are not calm. We are not tranquil. We are that which animates, that which glows. Hold us, and feel yourself re-align with the energy of Source. Use us to heal your gridwork, to rework your DNA, to channel your energies in more positive ways."

Apatite increases self-confidence and imagination, and opens your heart to Christ Consciousness. This is a good essence to support those who work in humanitarian fields. Physically, apatite can act as a hunger suppressant for those prone to over-eating or drinking, while it balances and re-aligns the chakras.

Aquamarine

Aquamarine, the stone of peace, can be used to help soothe wild or stressed animals and people. It also works on the throat chakra, increasing communication and diffusing anger.

Birds Eye Rhyolite

"See what we see. See to the core of things. See through the veil, through the drama, through the illusions of your reality and go deeply into your cellular makeup, into the energetic patterning of the world."

Birdseye Rhyolite helps you find your path and harness your full creative potential. Use it to see to the heart of issues for self-healing. Rhyolite helps us enjoy our work in life and encourages us to reach our goals.

Bloodstone

Bloodstone is one of my favorite grounding stones. Traditionally, it was believed that the dark green quartz stone received its red iron flecks from the blood of Christ at the crucifixion, rendering it capable of miracle healings. I have found that bloodstone is indeed a powerful healer, cleansing the blood, liver and reproductive systems, and it can be helpful in all dis-eases. It activates the root and heart chakras and draws energy from the earth directly through the legs and reproductive organs, dispersing energy equally throughout the entire body via the circulatory system and the meridians. It is a comforting, protective stone that brings calm and reassurance to the wearer, lowering the heart rate and blood pressure while soothing the soul.

Boji Stones/ Kansas Pop Rocks

Boji stones come from the base of a natural pyramid-shaped hill in at the heart of the United States in Kansas, and help to center and balance the individual. They can be bought and used in pairs, one female and one male, to balance yin and yang energy. The female stones generally have smooth surfaces, and the males rough. They direct excess energy into the earth and help keep the holder rooted on earth, in the physical. Boji stones can be used with great success to bring people "back to earth" when they get too flighty or spacey, and help counteract excess or disruptive geopathic and environmental energies.

Calcite

Calcite is a gentle, friendly stone that helps clear disturbances in energy fields be they geopathic, electromagnetic, or in the body. Use calcite to clear your energy when you feel you are picking up to much energy from people around you, or when you are over-stimulated. Calcite comes in many colors and opacities, but the clear or translucent varieties are best for this purpose. Calcite with rainbows in it triggers miraculous change. Yellow and honey calcite are both fantastic for use in healing work, whereas orange calcite can lift the energy in a room. Try working with the various colors calcite comes in – it is a good beginning for those unfamiliar with crystal work, due to its soothing, gentle manner.

Carnelian

This is another of my favorite grounding stones. I consider carnelian indispensible to anyone working with other people on a healing basis. This beautiful reddish to brown stone helps facilitate a constant exchange of this energy with the earth, allowing the wearer to become one with her surroundings. Negativity rolls off the back when one bears this stone, making the bearer impervious to ill will from others. It helps heal wounds of the heart and body. Carnelian energizes the physical body and stimulates healthful activity while grounding. Excess energy from the upper chakras is transmuted by carnelian into physical strength and vitality. This is a fantastic stone for anyone who is feeling bullied or weak in any way. It helps heal wounds of the heart, blood and body.

Celestobarite

"We will help you, and thus all who come in contact with you, raise your vibration and release all your fears forever. Yes, that's right, we said forever. We are extremely powerful yet relatively gentle tool that shows you exactly what is remaining in your way as an obstacle to your spiritual development, and allows you to move past these obstacles with ease and contentment. And the energetic effects of us becomes permanently lodged in your aura, so that everyone who comes near you also begins to feel a similar shift, and then this energy remains imprinted in them, affecting others, and so on, and so on. In this way, you literally shift the entire world. Are you ready? There is no pressure

here – all will be easy and well. You shall experience contentment and a joyful flow to your life as never before. Here we go!"

Special note: Celestobarite elixirs should be made using the indirect method.

Chlorite in Quartz

"We are green and white and love-Green for the heart, white for the Angels...the Angels of healing and love-We heal all things we are near-We give energy hugs because hugs are so wonderful-Companionship, love, joy in one's self and others-Relationship builders-Get rid of old relationship matters and move on no matter what type-We are here for love, we speak and work for love-Expand your heart and grow happiness with it-Love the small things in life. The small little joys, the gentle moments-The small joys will become larger & larger when you expand your heart-Most people don't realize how closed their hearts are-Society does that to us...don't trust this person, or be wary of that-In the higher realms there is no reason for fear-We are all moving towards the higher realms-Rejoice in your being and the journey you're on-What reason do you have not to?-There is no place for fear and discontent in the higher realms-Get rid of it, don't dwell on it, and it will cease to exist-You CAN create your own happiness-We help you move closer to that ability-We all have it, we help you find where you put it-We are done, thank you"

Chlorite is a purifier and a cleanser for the aura, chakras and meridians. It is very powerful at eliminating toxins and deep-rooted illnesses or miasms from the body – drink lots of water when you use this crystal to support your detoxification process.

Chrysocolla

"We open the door. We let in the light. We help you heal your self, we are the physician's stone, a stone of regeneration and energy. We activate the thymus gland and remind your body that it can live forever. You can live forever. This is real. This is the ability of your human body, to live and experience as long as you wanting and desiring to live and to be in this vessel. So often, you choose to begin anew, to begin fresh, forgetting that your body has the potential to refresh itself. You do not need to be reborn. You have the power to rebirth your self here, now. This is the truth, for we are the truth bearers."

Some people call Chrysocolla the "Peace Crystal" due to its ability to calm and soothe the mind. Chrysocolla is a gentle stone, unleashing its healing powers upon the powers slowly so that your psyche and physical body can acclimate smoothly to its healing powers. Due to its copper content, Chrysocolla is a wonderful stone for channeling energies and cleaning the aura, releasing toxic emotions and stress from all layers of the body. It helps you reach into your inner well of strength and fortitude.

Chrysocolla is very stabilizing and fortifying, and a wonderful stone to use around the home or office to improve communication and relationships. Place it in upon your altar to help you attract a mate or lover. Some people like to combine it with copper wrapping to further increase Chrysocolla's abilities. It is also believed by many to help foster wealth and increase good fortune.

Native American shamans used Chrysocolla to boost the immune system and soothe patients. Indeed, it is known to help benefit rational, clear thinking, and is often used by public speakers boost confidence. Crystal healers place Chrysocolla directly on body to lower blood pressure; treat infections, fever, and pain; and detoxify the liver.

Due to its high copper content, chrysocolla is best infused in elixirs via the indirect method.

Chrysoprase

This stone harnesses the supreme powers of love and forgiveness, connecting you directly to the compassion of Buddha and the Christ. Use Chrysoprase for all heart chakra healing and to raise your vibrational alignment. Very good for inspiring loyalty and fidelity.

Citrine

Need a smile? Give citrine a try – it's hard to frown when this stone is around. Citrine lets in the light of day. Access the power of the sun, and all its associated deities. Citrine is wonderful for clearing dark, heavy energy from the home or body. It opens the third chakra and heals digestive issues. Traditionally, it is used to attract wealth and prosperity.

Creedite

"Vibrating in the same light ray as citrine, we connect the roots of your self-confidence and joy to your heart chakra, allowing you to truly let happiness and abundance into the core of your being and soul. We help you feel more confident and strong, uplifting not only your own energy layers of being but letting your light radiate to those around you, creating harmony and bliss wherever you go."

Creedite aligns your upper chakras, allowing you to be more in tune with your higher self. This alignment fosters feeling of joy, happiness and relaxation. Use of creedite during meditation allows messages to come through with more clarity and for the higher good. It helps one access the Akashic records and past life information.

Physically, creedite helps to body simulate vitamins A, E, and B, and is helpful during liver cleanses.

Please Note: Creedite contains aluminum. Make your essences safely using the indirect infusion method.

Danburite

Whether we spend too much time in our upper chakras and out of our bodies, or our souls are still not sure that incarnating was the best idea, danburite helps us feel more comfortable in our bodies and brings us back to reality while facilitating an open channel to our higher selves. The pink pieces have a particularly soothing effect, though all danburite is calming.

Diamond

Diamonds really can be your best friend. Diamonds are extremely resilient and loyal in nature. They inspire feelings of security and fidelity, and tend to raise the vibration of all they come in contact with. It is certainly no mistake that they have become so intertwined with the traditions of marriage and romance in much of the world.

Dunite, aka (Olivine Peridotite)

"We are in the family of Peridot, but we carry a slightly different vibration. We allow the energy centers of the solar plexus and third chakras to merge and flow with ease into the heart center. We bring in more protection and grounding energy than the more commonly used peridot, thus allowing for fuller, more complete feelings of forgiveness and closure with past issues where blame, anger and guilt have been stored in the lower chakras. We allow these issues to rise to the surface and be transmuted by the light of love."

Dunite is an invaluable tool for maintaining balance when all around you is triggering you. Dunite forms a protective auric shield around your body and stabilizes the chakras. Before you use Dunite it is important that you balance and align all your chakras and it will maintain them in whatever state they are in. Dunite, as part of the peridot family, naturally heals the heart and solar plexus chakras, fostering openness and acceptance in relationships while it clears anger, guilt and jealousy.

In the physical, try using Dunite to improve your vision, digestion, circulation and heart. It acts as a general tonic, releasing toxins, and strengthening and regenerating the body. Emotionally, it relieves stress and is helpful for bipolar disorder.

Emerald

"We are the lightworkers of the crystal world, the healers of the heart, the ones who open the body to all the energies of the soul. Wear us, and you will be infused with the power of source. Wear us, and feel the fullness of your momentum and capability for creation. You are a powerhouse. We supply the fuel, we tune up your engine, we rev you up.

Tap in to the green ray of light healing, and reconnect with wonder and joy."

As a green stone, emerald is connected to the heart chakra and considered a "stone of love". In Asia it is associated with Quan Yin, the goddess of compassion and mercy. In Rome it was associated with Mercury, the God of messages and travel, and was carried travelers for protection. Early Christians wore it to show their faith and belief.

Emerald has a long history of use for healing and protection. It was carried in workshops by ancient artisans to improve their eyesight, placed over the heart to protect one from demonic possession, and believed to heal digestive disorders. Modern crystal healers use emerald to open the heart chakra and improve a variety of mood and stress disorders, as well as treat pain and back issues. Emeralds are extremely powerful, high vibration stones. They soothe the nervous system while strengthening and invigorating the body.

Emeralds can vary in coloration. The blue-green emeralds are considered more Yin, while the warmer yellow-greens are more yang. Light green emeralds are considered the most highly attuned with psychic, spiritual matters, and darker emeralds are believed to be more calming and physically healing. To recharge your stone, wash it with cool water and place near a ruby, quartz or diamond.

As with all green stones, emeralds can be used to encourage growth, fertility and abundance. This may be applied to the home, work, garden or one's own body. It is cooling, and may be helpful placed near those with traumatic injuries or burns. Try making a gem elixir of this stone with water to soothe eyestrain, treat pain and promote general healing and immunity.

Epidote

"We will bring you the balance and serenity which so many are seeking. We help you cool off tempers while strengthening your inner resources. A still river, our waters run deep: do not underestimate the power of epidote to carry you to new and exciting places in a short amount of time, safely and surely, we will deliver you."

Epidote is a stone of increasing energies. It has a tendency to increase anything it touches, whether the thing it touches is energy or a material object. As such, it is quite helpful both for growing businesses and souls. It is a stone that enhances emotional and spiritual growth by clearing repressed emotions and raising vibrations.

Epidote is very good at helping us get through difficult times, as it helps decrease sadness, grief, anger and panic by cleansing the emotional body while clearing energy blockages in the physical and subtle bodies. It is very beneficial in any work with tumors or growths.

Fun Fact: The green color found in Unakite is inclusions of Epidote

Eudialyte

Eudialyte is a stone that allows you to GROW. It releases your fears which hold you back, and your fear of fears, too. It helps to ground your desires in reality and bring them to fruition in a balanced manner that blends joyful creation with logic and mass consciousness. It helps you to rationalize everything you want in a way that helps you to attain it more quickly and fully.

Physically, Eudialyte helps thyroid and pancreatic issues, and opens Kundalini pathways. It is known to amplify the Alpha brain wave pattern during the creative state as well as the dream state, and some healers like to use it for clearing residual souls (ghosts) from the physical plane. It is very helpful in any work with the terminally ill.

Fairy Cross, or Staurolite

"We are called fairy crosses, but really we are so much more than that. Use us to connect to the fae if you wish – but we are here to connect you to the entire to earth, to all beings sentient in your dimension and beyond to who you are connected already through your energy patterning and even your DNA. We are as magnets, who will draw to you a greater connectivity with all that is, all that was, and all that will be. Use us to draw to you that which you are wanting. Be very careful – don't think about the things you do not want when you are using us, for we cannot tell the difference! We merely hear your frequency, and amplify it. In all ways, for all times. We are of the universe. We are everything. We are all all all all. Use us wisely, and do not be afraid!"

Staurolite has been know for centuries as a good luck talisman, and many believed that it could protect the wearer against witchcraft, illness and physical harm. President Theodore Roosevelt and President Wilson, Thomas A. Edison, Colonel Charles Lindbergh, and may royal persons of carried this stone on a regular basis. One legend tells that Staurolite healed Richard the Lionhearted of malaria during his Crusades in the Middle East.

Staurolite represents the four elements and joining of spirit with earth/matter. It can be used to connect the physical, astral and spiritual parts of oneself to heighten your vibration and increase your presence in the here and now.

Physically, Staurolite is used by healers to strengthen one's connection to the physical body.

Fire Agate

"We are grounding and energizing. We bring in all the creative power of the universe to you on the powerful arc of the rainbow. We are the voice of source. We are the mind of the angels. We are the power of the earth. We are YOU. We are now, only in the now, and we will help you to find your true center."

Fire agate increases strength and courage, bringing a deep sense of calm and security. It is a very strong grounding and protection stone. As a fire stone, it opens the base chakra, stimulates energy flow, and enhances sexuality and creativity.

Physically it heals the stomach, nervous, endocrine systems, strengthens night vision and reduces hot flashes (contrary to what one might guess!) Metaphysical healing lore professes that fire agate enhances all healing energies, and assists with healing of the circulatory system, lymph system, and intestines.

Fluorite

"We are here to bring you balance. In your ever changing world, during ever changing times, we will balance and harmonize the waters that flow through your body. The more your vibration rises, the more susceptible you are to the energies that surround you, the frequencies that are emitted by the technology of your present reality, by ley lines, by

organisms. We keep your own frequency tuned. We keep it humming as it should, the molecules of your physical reality aligned with the harmonies emitted from source. We help your cells ring with the sounds of angels, with the love of god, of all that is."

Fluorite is a fantastic stone for clearing and balancing excess energy, while facilitating psychic opening and growth. It is a healing stone for the heart and the mind. It regulates the flow of energy into the upper body and allows it to pass through the torso to the legs, making it easier to ground. It works very well with selenite to clear negativity from the environment, and worn with black tourmaline will allow the kundalini to flow easily through the entire body. Place a large piece in the center of a room or each corner of a house to eliminate geopathic stress.

Fuchsite

"We hold the essence of all-one-peace within its shining form. We are intricately connected to the overlighting angels and nature devas of your world, and as such we can connect you with the PEACE that is your divine birthright. Let us smooth the rough edges from your day, let us sooth your spirit and show you how to just be. To be in the moment, to be at one with all moments, all the time, always, never rushing, never worried, that is the gift of fuchsite, the divine all-one state of being that will benefit humanity more than any other lesson ever could."

Fuchsite enhances the power of other minerals and is a great stone to use during healing sessions because it will increase energy transfer when multiple stones are used for healing. It has been linked by other crystal healers to Archangel Raphael, the angel of heart healing. Fuchsite activates our connection to nature, including the nature devas and faeries. Since it cleanses and protects the auric fields of everyone who is near it, fuchsite further encourages communication with animals and nature spirits.

Physically, fuchsite is a stabilizing mineral for people who have challenges with balancing blood sugar levels, ADHD, or mood swings. The use of fuchsite crystal essence is a great remedy for these situations. Simply take a few drops after each meal or throughout the day to decrease your severe highs and lows. It is also known to benefit red and white blood cell counts, and ameliorate spinal issues.

Garnet

Deep, dark red garnet is very similar to bloodstone in its properties, with its healing effect more focused on the blood and sexual organs rather than the entire body. It has the further effect of enhancing sexuality and virility, and is one of the best stones to awaken and open the root chakra. It is a good healing stone for those who desire love and intimacy, but also fear it.

Granite

Heat and shock resistant, granite is happy to lend us its strength and help us connect with the earth. Food prepared on granite countertops often tastes fresher, and it has the power to help transmute pesticides used on non-organic crops. Place your hands on the countertop and take a few deep breaths, letting your frustrations of the day be cleared and the good strong energy of the granite infuse you.

Hematite

"Shield yourself. This is the message you receive all the time from your ego. You are always thinking about how to protect yourselves from other people, from disaster, from your fears. We show you there is nothing to fear. It is not that we are protective, as so many of you say, but that we remove the fear and the perceived need for self-preservation which so many of you feel at so many moments during your lives. We return you to the simple state of just being and acting, how you were as a child before you were taught the rules and told "don't do this", "don't do that," "now's not the time." It's always the time. It is always right. You have NOTHING to fear. Truly. You can do and be whatever you want. So smile. Show your appreciation and your happiness to everyone around you. Smile at your enemies. Smile at your friends. Smile at the sun, moon and stars. Smile, and be radiant, and be delighted and delight-full. We are a mirror of truth; we reflect your soul-smile, your true face, back to you so that you can really live."

Hematite is a form of iron oxide that is harder than pure iron. Its name comes from the Greek word for blood, as its unpolished form can oxidize to a deep blood red. It tends to be most frequently associated with the base chakra, although I feel that it is highly attuned with the silver rays of the crown chakra. Many find it to be quite grounding and protective, due to its tendency to help us feel safe and increase our life energies. It is known as a stone for the mind, often being used to enhance memory and concentration.

As a slightly magnetized stone, hematite helps to align the polarities in our bodies, connecting our meridians and augmenting our own geo-magnetic alignments. It helps to balance our body, mind and spirit, connecting all our chakras from the base up through our crown chakra to our higher selves.

It is a very strong, energized stone, and some people can find it a bit difficult to work with. If you have a hard time letting go, hematite might be a bit of a challenge for you since it overrides the fears of the ego with the delights and confidence of the soul. It is often characterized as a very yang, male stone, but actually I feel that hematite is simply source. Neither male nor female, simply power without sex or predisposition.

Physically, hematite helps restore circulation and increase red blood cell production. It is beneficial for structural, physical issues of all kinds, from scarring to tears to wounds and breaks.

Cleanse hematite regularly by the light of the sun or moon. Avoid washing or directly infusing hematite in water due to its high iron content and potential for oxidation.

Hemimorphite

"We have been waiting. We have been watching. We are clear. We are bright. We harness the light and the energy and we shine it all around us. We show you the way through the darkest night, through the brightest light. We illuminate the shadows and show you the way. We are pure. We are bright."

Hemimorphite activates the chakras in the body and opens your higher chakras to the light of source. It wants to help us reach our full potential. Calming and relaxing, it opens the body to the spirit of forgiveness and peace. It allows us to remain in balance and appreciate all our emotions as creative expressions of life energy. Hemimorphite is believed to be activated by touch, instantly attuning to the bearer and becoming stronger the more it is used.

It is considered a very high vibration stone with strong protection and healing abilities. It helps us disconnect from our earth-bound ego, dissolve negative emotional patterns and gain greater confidence. Use it to combat insecurity issues, sadness or depression. It is a wonderful stone for those searching for inner peace and is helpful to those who would work as psychic channels.

Physically, hemimorphite is used by crystal healers to balance hormones and heal dis-ease in the chest and head. It is also said to help bring out our inner beauty and relieve pain.

Indicolite

"We connect you to the mysteries of your soul. We are helpful for all inner and outer seeking, for adventures within and without. With quartz, we allow you to see and hear its messages even more clearly, with the quartz acting a sort of intermediary or interpreter between our human physical minds and the extremely high source vibration of the indigo ray. We will clear out your oldest, deepest and darkest patterns, and help lift you into the higher realms. This is a good place to start, a good place to begin your transformation into the best and the brightest stars that you already are."

Indicolite is the rarest color of tourmaline, its present name deriving from an older name of "indigolite" referring to its desirable dark blue color. It will clear all chakras, but especially resonates with the throat and third eye chakras. Because of its beneficial effect of the thymus and thyroid glands, it increases immune function and boosts healing powers throughout the physical and energy bodies.

It enhances harmonic resonance and feelings of peace, and is a wonderful stone for decreasing pain. Under your pillow, indicolite can help enhance sleep and dreaming.

Jasper

Jasper is a widely varying stone and comes in many colors which offer slight modifications to its energy. Overall, jasper is a grounding, strengthening and relaxing stone. It is a form of quartz, and helps gently raise one's vibration while keeping one firmly rooted in the physical realms. It is a stone made to help you adjust to planet Earth – especially good for the young, old, and infirm due to its boosting, uplifting properties.

Jet

Jet is well known as a low-cost, attractive jewelry stone. Like diamond, it is popular with good reason. Jet is very protective, grounding and balancing. It gives the wearer a sense of self-confidence and assurance – always good in a fine piece of jewelry! It is organic in origin, a sort of fossilized wood. Some people even call it "black amber" although jet does not come from the resin of trees, but rather the wood itself. Among many cultures worldwide, jet has long been associated with the Gods and the dead. It is believed to help heal deep emotions such as sadness and grief, and physical ailments stemming from said emotional issues.

Kunzite

"We are a master healer stone. We are one of the key stones for ascension into the New Age. Every color variation, every specimen, has something invaluable to teach you humans. Every piece no matter how small or imperfect will raise your vibration. Use us well, for that is the only way one can use Kunzite. No ill may come of this stone. No harm, no bad thought or feelings. Only love, compassion, gentle strength and healing."

Kunzite is a powerful, high level stone. It is a super heart stone, opening you to Christ Consciousness, Buddha Compassion and God-Love. It helps you empathize with others and forgive the past. It is very self-healing, helping you remove pressure from yourself and release blocks that are preventing your from progressing on your life journey.

Kunzite calms the nervous system and soothes the mind, making it invaluable for treating panic attacks and a host of psychiatric disorders.

Kyanite

"Black. Blue. Green. Orange. White. Gray. We all work the same. We all align the waters in your body so that your energies can flow properly. We allow the meridians to connect, the chakras to flow, and your mind and body to be fully open and receptive to the intentions of your true self, your own source energy. We facilitate balance and flow. Nothing more. Nothing less. When you are balanced, you are able to manifest all that you want and need, and see your path most clearly. When you are flowing, you are joyful and easy, and the world flows with you."

The name "Kyanite" derives from the Greek word for deep blue, *kyanos*. It is a silicate mineral characterized by a diamond-like cleavage in one direction and two separate hardnesses, making it a challenging stone to cut or facet. Kyanite clears and aligns the chakras of all those who come near it. When it is worn, it has a constant protective and grounding effect as it clears and aligns the chakras, clears and aligns the energy systems of the body, over and over again. The bearer of this stone is quite difficult to knock off-balance energetically. Because the chakras are aligned and open, one's higher self and energy body are able to enter the physical body, leading to higher ascension and attunements. Qi and kundalini energies flow better throughout the entire body when kyanite is around. Because it enhances energy flow and calms the central nervous system, it promotes feelings of tranquility and peace.

Kyanite is easily found in many shades of blue and green, as well as orange and black: black Kyanite is considered more protective but less aligning than blue Kyanite, while the green focuses its healing energy more on the physical body. Regardless of its color, Kyanite is able to attune the wearer to his or her true path, opening channels of creativity, dreaming and visualization.

Physically, Kyanite can assist in pain management and glandular disorders. It is also believed to be effective against fevers and infections because it helps return the body to its natural state of perfection.

Labradorite, a.k.a Spectrolite

Labradorite is a high vibration stone filled with an inner energy and light that literally flashes and radiates through the bearer. It brings all chakras and layers of the body into alignment. It refines DNA, and allows your soul to feel more comfortable within the confines of its physical body and this dimensional reality. When the physical and spiritual aspects of yourself are in harmony it is easier to remain calm and peaceful, secure in your own true self, you can meet the day with assurance and ease. Labradorite is often used to balance issues of both the 1st, 6th and 7th chakras – parts of the body regulating the mind, digestion, sexuality and circulation.

Lapis Lazuli

"We were the stone of the gods. We were used to access immense amounts of electrical power by the ancients, and later shamans used us successfully to create an open dialogue with the powers that be. Use us to tap into ALL that IS. Use us to bring new levels of wealth and harmony into your life. We can align you to your Divine Blueprint, with your True Path, the Path with a Heart, the life you are wanting and meant to be living. Many of you are close, so close already. We will bring you closer."

Lapis has been highly valued for many thousands of years, and almost every culture has used lapis in some way to access the gods through magical ceremonies and decorate holy places. Lapis forms a sphere of protection around the upper chakras and filters psychic noise, helping induce peace and relaxation. As it helps you identify your inner truth, it amplifies honesty and compassion within both the conscious and subconscious mind. It's a wonderful stone to use when studying or preparing for public speaking.

Physically, lapis may be used to lower blood pressure and boost thymus activity. Use lapis to fight depression, insomnia and nervous dispositions.

Larimar

"We bring you both the calm and power of the sea. The calm: the knowing that every tide out brings a tide in, the interconnectedness of all that dwell in the water, the cellular healing ability of the salted mineral waters. The power: the great waves that can wash away an island, the ability to mold rock and dissolve metal, the creative essence of the earth and all her fury. We can help you make peace in the middle of a storm. We hold the knowledge of the earth's oldest history, the origin of your species, the story of all who have come before. We are the womb of your mother, the essence of your father. We are a stone of deep answers, and soothing wisdom."

Larimar is especially tuned with the 5th chakra in the throat area of the body. Use it with Lapis to help regulate thyroid and thymus gland malfunction, or to support general healing and communication. Associated as it is with the sea, Larimar helps regulate the element of water in the body. It supports the natural energetic ebb and flow, and helps dissolve blockages that may cause cellular dysfunction. It opens the mind and helps ease emotional stress.

Leopardskin Jasper

This particular jasper allows one to get in touch with animals and the forest/jungle aspect of the earth. It facilitates animal communication and shapeshifting, which is essentially the transmutation of one's higher purpose within the physical. It

151

allows the manifestation of one's will on the earthly plane. It calls in the protection of large cats to the wearer, and allows one to become one with one's surroundings and the earth, making it easier to ground.

Lepidolite

"Lepidolite flows directly with Source. See those sparkles? That is a physical representation of source. Wherever there is sparkle, you are invoking source love, source light, source creation. Lepidolote helps you tap in directly to the angels, god and the ascended masters. It connects you to all that is divine, all that is true, all that is you. It balances your chakras and enacts your ability to walk as a god upon the earth. Claim your birthright. Be divine."

Also known as "Peace stone" and "Lilalite" (Playful Stone), lepidolite is a form of mica discovered in the 1700s in the Czech Republic. The purple and pink mineral is also found in Brazil, Africa and the United States. Its color derives from lithium, which is no surprise when one considers the calming effect of this stone.

Lepidolite clears away negative energies and raises your vibration. It helps soothe the mind and body by connecting you with Source energy and Source love. Many people find it helpful to use during meditation and astral travel, because it is so adept at connecting us to our higher self. It can also be used to access the Akashic records or facilitate channeling. Use it to clear obstacles and create a new life.

Lepidolite combines well with rose quartz to help heal relationships, and is very nice used at night to create a restful atmosphere and induce deep sleep. It is deeply harmonizing and balancing. Use it to ameliorate grief and the emotional effects of trauma or abuse.

Physically, it is believed to help detoxify the body and heal DNA. It may be used to clear electromagnetic disturbances and calm the energy in a room. Because of its soothing effect, it is often recommended in cases of psychiatric imbalance or nerve disorders. It is also said to strengthen the immune system and help with allergies.

Malachite

Malachite is an excellent for general physical healing. It helps boost all manner of creative processes, both material and spiritual, from personal finances to physical fertility. Because malachite is high in copper, it is not recommended to place this stone in drinking water. Use the indirect method of infusion or use green agate, which has very similar properties.

Moonstone

Moonstone is a quiet, introspective stone. It increases one's ability to dream and hear one's own inner thoughts. It is, indeed, connective strongly to the moon and the tides, and helps us "go with the flow." Use moonstone to clear negativity from your surroundings and protect you during travel over water. Physically, moonstone is often used to benefit female disorders and as a sleep aide.

Morganite

"Harness the healing power of love. We induce a warm a feeling of self-love all around you, and help instill confidence and serenity in the bearer. We help others to see you in the full light of your soul-ness, and enable you to do the same."

Morganite is a rare pink member of the Beryl family, the same family as Aquamarine and Emerald. It is a fantastic stone for those working on love and trust issues. It helps you open up and accept blessings as they come your way. It helps you live in the moment and feel secure in the idea that life is change – and isn't it grand? Morganite removes self-doubt and self-imposed fears so that you can embrace your true, most wonderful, self.

If you are feeling sad or abandoned, morganite will help lift you up with the power of self-love. Many people associate morganite with angels, although really what it does is connect you to ALL that is, to source energy. To you. It is a very high-frequency stone.

Physically, morganite can benefit many dis-eases, but is particularly aligned with the heart, thymus and lungs.

Nuumite

"Starchildren. Finally, you return. We watch you, we hear you, and now, you are beginning to hear us again, too. This stone you hold here is a communication stone, a means to contact we the races who seeded you there on Earth. Questions? We have many answers. We are mostly concerned with helping you to once again reach your fullest potentials, to raise your awareness and energies on earth so that you can emerge as a stronger, more compassionate race. We want your heart and souls to fly, and even your bodies. You have so many abilities you have

154

yet to tap into. But the beginning has been made, and we will lift you up further."

Nuummite is the oldest known mineral in existence at around 3 billion years old. It is a laminate mined north of Nuuk, Southern Greenland, in a high, difficult mountain terrain. It is volcanic in origin and its unique flash derives from millennia of pressing and metamorphism.

Nuummite has called both the Sorcerers and Magician's stone. It has strong elemental properties that can awaken magical abilities in those who align with it. At the very least, it carries a high vibration that tends to catalyze spiritual growth and personal improvement.

It can help you access past lives and times well beyond modern history. It has a potent electro-magnetic field and many healers use it to help clear obstacles and energy drains from the physical, auric and etheric bodies. Because of this, nuummite is also helpful in recovering lost memories and helping us overcome limitations we have placed upon ourselves.

Nuummite is strongly shielding and grounding, making it a wonderful stone for protection and fortitude. It clears the aura and aligns the chakras on all levels.

When you work a lot with Nuummite, lucky coincidences increase and you often begin to lead a sort of charmed life. This is part of the magic it imparts – a natural side-effect of being in tune with your true self.

Obsidian, or Apache Tears

Obsidian is one of the most grounding, protective stones you can find. Obsidian looks opaque, but is actually translucent, which helps allow us to see through the negativity to the positive, and vice versa, to see what is hidden. Apache Tears are a particular variety of obsidian that is steeped in legend, and has the added quality of helping one cope with issues of anger, grief, and forgiveness. Apache storytellers say that one day a group of Apaches was ambushed by an enemy tribe (recent versions have transmuted the tribe into a white man's cavalry) and in the fight they were cornered and forced over a cliff to their deaths. When the women found them, they wept long and hard, and as their tears struck the ground, each tear was transformed into small, round pieces of obsidian. When you carry an Apache Tear, legend says, you will never cry, for the women shed enough tears for all. (For an obsidian with gentler balancing properties, see **Snowflake Obsidian**.)

Onyx

Onyx can be found in many earthy colors, including brown, green, and black. Long used as a popular stone for men's jewelry, onyx has a warm, safe, feeling. The green can be mossy or brilliant, and is good for healing and connecting to nature. The deep emerald green variation is one of my favorite stones to wear in a ring. It has a high healing vibration and yet still carries the sense of protectiveness that all onyx bears. Brown onyx helps kundalini energy flow up and through the root chakra, and remediates many reproductive issues. Black onyx is the best of all onyx types for shielding one from negativity and lending the wearer courage and strength.

Petrified Wood

Petrified wood is not a stone, per se, but ancient wood which has fossilized over the millennia to form a light, stone like substance. Jet is a form of black, petrified wood that has been used in jewelry for centuries. All petrified wood helps root us to the earth while filtering out toxic thoughts and patterns from our DNA, much as live plants filter and purify the air and water, which passes through them.

Prehnite

This light minty green to blue stone can often be found among gray gravel driveways, roads and ditches in the Northeastern United States. It is considered very protective, while also stimulating energy flow throughout the body. I find it to be quietly uplifting, allowing the heart chakra to open and unfold and help facilitate enhanced spiritual communication, meditation and astral travel.

Quartz

Quartz is a silicate mineral in the form of a silicon oxygen tetrahedron. It is energizing, clearing and strengthening, and can be used to empower any healing remedy. It is found in large quantities throughout the Earth, in combination with many other stones and minerals. This is not a coincidence: quartz amplifies and harmonizes the energies of other stones. Quartz, whether clear or white, can be used for practically any purpose. If there is a stone you would really like to work with, but you can't find or afford it, try asking a piece of quartz to align with the energy of that stone and be used in its place (make sure you ask first – some pieces may not want to "play dress-up".) Quartz is used in clocks, computers and various electronic devices as a short term memory processor and timekeeper. It has the ability to store short transient signals in the form of a short delay circuit. IBM scientists have, in recent years, achieved technological breakthroughs using silicate crystals to create extremely fast computer processors. There are a myriad of quartz forms on the market: natural, shaped, points, chunks, and much more. Some connect you to ancient civilizations, some are attuned for healing work, some are said to help increase your intuition or wealth. As with all stones, use your intuition. Follow your heart, follow your joy. Choose the stone that speaks to you, that brings a smile to your face.

Rose Quartz

Rose Quartz is well-known for its loving qualities. It is a very gentle, peaceful stone that quietly uplifts the aura and soothes the mind. Rose Quartz is particularly wonderful for any sort of work with children; it helps them feel cherished and protected. It has a warm, positive yin quality. Use rose quartz to heal or open the heart chakra, encourage forgiveness and allow the release of anger and unhappiness.

Ruby

Ruby is a powerful, sensual stone. It is intrinsically aligned with the root chakra, connecting all the lower chakras up to the heart chakra so that one can live a grounded life with an open heart. Ruby raises the vital life force of the physical body and encourages kundalini or Qi energy to run properly. It allows us to access our true desires and release inhibitions, unblocking our path to enjoyment and fulfillment here in the physical plane of existence. It helps remove anger and dissatisfaction from the equation. Physically, ruby is especially beneficial to the reproductive and hormonal systems

Ruby with Kyanite

"Clear the path to universal Christ Consciousness. You have opened your hearts, now let us help you hollow them out, refresh them and make them as new and as pure as the heart of the universe. Let the center of your being being filled with the light of Source. We are here to help you be the true you."

Ruby and Kyanite together is a powerhouse combination that helps manifest dreams in a manner that benefits the highest good of all involved. It keeps you balanced, clearing negativity while raising your life energies. In this way it is supremely nurturing, encouraging positive emotions and open heart.

Selenite, or White Gypsum

"Selenite was placed here on earth by the angels. We have been used by mankind for millennia to clear the burdens of physical being, to realign the spiritual being at the center of your body and to raise your vibration. We facilitate astral projection and allow the physical body to transcend your current earthly realm to reach higher dimensions."

Selenite is an amazing stone, perhaps one of the most powerful and indispensible stones in a healer's arsenal. Passed through the aura and around the body, selenite will cut cords and remove energy drains. Placed in a room it will clear geopathic and electromagnetic stress, as well as any other form of negativity. It is so good at clearing that the stone itself never needs to be cleansed, as it will never hold negative energy itself. It is amazing when held in the hand and passed over the body as a scanning device – it helps you to better sense areas which need attention and then to direct your healing energy toward the client. It is, in essence, the perfect hollow tube which shamanic elders such as Fools Crow so often spoke of.

Selenite increases peace and calm around it. It helps us access past lives, and then remove any blockages or negativity left over from the experience that may be tainting this life. Many people like to use the stone for psychic amplification due to its ability to transmit light and energy as it aligns and clears the physical, auric and etheric bodies. Physically, it is often used in increasing spinal alignment.

Note: Do not wash or immerse selenite, it is mildly water-soluble and will slowly degrade.

Shaman Stones/Moqui Balls

Shaman stones, or moqui balls, are found in the Moqui Desert. Balls of sandstone coated with iron ore, they are believed to have formed when a giant meteor struck the earth and flash-melted the iron present in the sand. They are prized for their ability to help facilitate meditative states and trance journeys while still keeping one linked to their physical body. Both alien and terrestrial, shaman stones offer an unusual link between realities and dimensions. Due to their strong magnetic vibration, they present an ideal anchor to those who would travel between different planes of realities, so that one can easily return to one's body and time. Once through with trance work, shaman stones are also quite helpful for re-connecting to the physical realm and clearing one's head.

Shiva Lingham Stones

Shiva Lingham stones are oblong stones from the holy Narmada River in India, naturally formed into an egg-like shape by eons of water flow, and then further smoothed by the hands of man. In India it is believed that these stones are direct links to Shiva and the fiery pillar of creation, and when you hold these stones in your hands, you are holding the power of the god Shiva in your hands. Remember India Jones & The Temple of Doom? That was a radiant Shiva Lingham stone the village lost. These stone are indeed considered holy in India, and are believed to unify feminine and masculine energy into creative harmony. Use them to activate the root chakra and heal sexual and reproductive organs. A Shiva Lingham placed in a bedroom encourages passion; held in meditation, it creates a strong connection with both the creative energies of the feminine and with male potency. It is a powerful stone for willful manifestation. In our own healing circles at Earth Lodge, we have found that one large shiva lingham placed at the foot of each leg of the massage table helps connect all our energies to each other – our healing energy flows more freely from our circle of hands to the person laying on the table, down to the earth and channeling source. We often use various crystals under the table, changing them from week to week, person to person, but the shiva linghams have become a permanent fixture.

Shungite

"We are immortal. We are shungite. We hold old, old knowledge. That which you have hidden away or try to deny we can see, we know. Would you like to see what is hidden? We can help you with that. Let us help clear out the cobwebs, bring the darkness to light, and illuminate your being, your life, your world."

Shungite is one of the oldest minerals in the world, contains almost every element in the period table and is noted for its unique carbon structure. It is known to exist only in Karelia, Russia, near Shunga lake, and is about 2 billion years old. Scientists argue over whether it was formed volcanically, from primitive microscopic organisms or via meteorite impact. Its appearance is similar to coal, but its age predates almost all life on earth and therefore other coal formations. It has been used for decades in Russia with verifiable scientific proof that it cleanses impurities and radiation from water and increases the bioavailability of water to the body. It has been shown that shungite has both filtrative and antibacterial action and is biologically active. It is said to cleanse water of various chlorine compounds, nitrates, copper, magnesium, and iron while enriching the water in potassium. Stones used in water enhancement should be cleansed by sunlight on a weekly basis and replaced every 6 months.

The majority of Shungite's healing power comes from its carbon components, fullerenes. American scientists identified the unique fullerenes in Shungite which have implications for nanotechnology and cancer therapies, and they received a Noble Prize for this discovery. Shungite infused in water releases fullerenes which enter our bodies and become extremely powerful antioxidants. Shungite enhanced water has also been show to greatly decrease the activity of histamines in the bloodstream, thereby reducing inflammation and helping those who suffer from allergies. Fullerenes are being researched by many manufacturers for their potential applications, including UV skin protection, solar arrays, radiation treatments, asthma treatments and nanotechnology.

Metaphysically, shungite is believed to work on all levels of your being -- the spiritual, mental, emotional, and physical bodies – and clear out all harmful elements. Shungite takes issues which are lurking in the etheric and astral planes and brings them to light, facilitating personal growth and enlightenment. It is extremely protective and lends feelings of safety to all those who work with it. Need a shield? Employ shungite.

Silicon

Silicon comprises over 90% of the earth's crust, but almost never occurs naturally in its absolute pure crystalline form. It is often synthesized in labs for use in modern technology, however, and may be obtained for personal use at some mineral shows or stores. This is a wonderful thing! Silicon speeds the body's transformation to a higher level of vibrational existence while repairing and optimizing DNA and RNA. In turn, it catalyzes and improves evolution. Many lightworkers insist that humanity is evolving into a crystalline, silicon-based physical body. When you work directly with silicon, this certainly feels true on a very basic level. Silicon is tremendously uplifting and energizing. How wonderful it would be to incorporate that feeling into a regular facet of mass consciousness, of regular human existence.

Slate

Slate is an old, old stone and soul, and brings us the wisdom of the ages. Its many layers allow us to read between the lines and find understanding on all levels. It contains the peace of the elderly, the knowledge that time has no bounds, and can bring that same peace and serenity to those who would work with it. A path of slate to your front door will wipe away the mundane cares and worries of all who tread it.

Smoky Quartz

Smoky Quartz is a dependable grounding stone that also carries clearing properties to open the crown chakra, allowing the dual energies of the earth and the higher realms to flow freely in and out of the body through both the crown and root chakras. It is a slow-moving healing stone, bringing elder knowledge and patience with it. When you are stressed or overloaded with mental energy, try holding a smoky quartz in your lap for a few minutes. Your breathing will slow, your heart rate will lower, and your mind will begin to know peace. Tibetan Smoky Quartz has the added benefit of carrying centuries of Buddhist prayer energy within it, helping to facilitate calm serenity in the face of adversity.

Snowflake Obsidian

Snowflake Obsidian is a sweet, friendly stone to use for protection and grounding. It will benefit almost anyone, but is particularly great for children or people with weak constitutions in place of the stronger protection stones such as black obsidian or hematite. Black with white "snowflake" marks, it seeks to balance yin and yang energy. It works with forgiveness to release anger and allows one to see both sides of things. It connects to both the lower and higher realms, without prejudice. Don't be fooled: despite its easy nature, snowflake obsidian contains great strength and is very, very shielding from negativity. This coupled with its gentle balancing nature make it a wonderful stone for young people to carry with them to school and play dates.

Soo Chow Marble

Soo Chow Marble from China contains a particularly calm, immovable spirit, more so than that of other marbles which are more likely to harbor the same high energy and sensitivities as the artists who often work with it. Soo Chow, on the other hand, immediately places one deep in the earth, her inner frequencies. This is the stone of the stoic dwarves of the path, the stone that moves time to keep pace with molasses. When you feel hurried or rushed, reach for Soo Chow. Feel your bonds to time release, for you are one with all.

Tektite

Tektites are very special. Tektite is always grounding and calming, a gift from above to connect you to the creative intent of your Planet. They can help you connect to your inner resources, and help you tap into all your true power and energies. Because it stimulates thought transmissions, meditation with a tektite can increase telepathy. Its vibrational energies have been known to heighten the awareness of its wearers, often by enhancing psychic sensitivity, clairaudient experiences and increasing the frequency of synchronicities in their lives. Many report having the experience of "seeing through the veil" of the physical world more readily with Tektite. It makes the hidden, deep truth obvious.

More than 2000 years ago, the Chinese referred to tektites as Inkstone of the Thundergod. Australian aborigines refer to them as Mabon, or 'magic' and believe that finding one brings good luck. In India, they are known as the Sacred Gem of Krishna. They assist one in attaining knowledge and learning lessons throughout the travels of life. Tektite from Tibet is believed to also carry the resonance of mantras, meditations and prayers that have been sung in that land for centuries. It carries some of the highest spiritual evolutionary energies on our Earth, and thus helps us tap into our highest potentialities.

Tiger's Eye

Tiger's eye re-organizes the energetic gridwork of the body so that we can function at our fullest ability. It is a very practical, strengthening stone, as well as protective and full of light. It is associated with the energies of the Sun, and will help alleviate darkness and sadness. It is a very good stone for children, especially those who could use a little extra attention or structure. Physically, Tiger's Eye is very good for the bones and vision problems.

Tiger Iron

"Are you ready to tap into all your strengths? Are you ready to be the true powerhouse of creation and decision that you are? Are you

ready to stop being bombarded by negative vibrations and begin having great days? Every day? Well, that is what we are here to help you with. We harness the power of gold and silver, the sun and the mirror, the light and the shield. We bring these powers straight into your being, into your blood, to become one with you. Talk to us, and we will talk to you. We will help show you the way to security and joy that you desire. We will light the fire in your soul. Do not be afraid. There is nothing to fear about this process. It will be easy. It will be great."

Tiger iron, also known as Mugglestone, blends the properties of three stones: hematite, red jasper, and golden tiger's eye. It is protective, stabilizing, and strengthening. It's good at increasing motivation and creativity, while boosting self-confidence. Physically, it is believed to improve the blood, muscles and bones.

Topaz

"We are a very high energy stone. We are similar to quartz in our healing potentials and versatility, but our energies are much, much more potent and focused. The vibrational powers of topaz shoot directly to the core of the physical and spiritual bodies, blasting through any barriers or indifferences. We are perfectly aligned with grid work because we can be charged for any purpose, regardless of our color, and once we are charged to a specific purpose our energies are unrelenting until the goal is reached. We are strong, empowering and of the highest vibration. Are you ready?"

Natural topaz crystals have the energy of soft, warm encouragement. Topaz is one of the hardest minerals, and is the hardest silicate mineral found in nature. Topaz helps foster empowerment, helping us heal ourselves and attain our dreams, always in a loving, joy-full way. Topaz is filled with positive source energy – negative emotions tend to disappear in its presence. It shows us the truth of all things, showing us the original good in all matters and allowing us to reach goals for the highest good of all involved.

For all its high energy, topaz is a naturally calming stone, helping smooth out the rough edges in ones psyche. Use it to heal headaches, digestive disorders and nerves.

Tourmaline

Tourmaline is not so very different from Topaz. It is another high energy stone that is quite soothing and positive in nature. It seems to be especially concerned with helping humanity evolve, and so will often allow you to get to the root of problems and negativity. When you use tourmaline in this way, it also helps you attain greater compassion and understanding, so that true healing may occur. Pink tourmaline and Watermelon tourmaline are further attuned to healing the heart chakra and opening us to greater amounts of unconditional love and Christ Energy.

Black tourmaline is a very grounding stone with high vibrations, and shields the wearer from negativity of all kinds, including electromagnetic waves and radiation. My favorite tourmaline specimens for grounding consist of the black rods at least the size of one's pinkie finger growing through clear or white quartz – they have a wonderfully clean effect on illnesses and the environment. It draws earth energy through the root chakra to increase one's vitality and energy.

Violet Obsidian

"We are the dream keepers, the holders of visions. We are the ones to call upon when your resolve is faltering, the ones to help you stay on your path. We are strength, we are beauty. We will help you to walk in the light and find your truth. There is nothing you can't do, there is no place you can't go or no one you cannot become. We are the dream keepers. Keep on keeping on."

Violet Obsidian is a rare variety of Obsidian that has the properties of the Third Eye, Crown and Higher Chakra energies. It is a very high vibration stone, showing us how to transmute fire into spirit. Use it to connect with your intuition and source energy, to help encourage dream recall and attain real spiritual growth. It is a nice, supportive stone for working with and clearing past lives and karmic attachments.

Unakite

Unakite is hands-down my favorite stone for working with issues of anger, guilt and forgiveness. It is a combination of pink feldspar, green epidote and colorless quartz, taking the qualities of each and creating a stone that will help heal your heart and open your soul to life again. If your heart chakra feels closed or walled off, give unakite a try. It is here to help you, it wants nothing more than to ease your pain and lift you up.

Harnessing the Power of the Earth

These days, many companies are selling earth energies made into vibrational remedies. These "environmental essences", as they are known in the industry, capture the vibration of specific places and physical events on the planet. An environmental essence might harness the energy of the aurora borealis or the imprint of a specific lunar eclipse. It might be useful to attune you with a particularly powerful ley line or holy place, or imbue you with the creative powers of a volcano.

While there are obviously countless remedies that can be made, in this chapter we will focus on some of the most common earth phenomena and their possible uses. When you approach a location to make an earth essence, remember that all locations on earth are under the domain of devas or nature spirits. Each deva has its own personality and energy signature, and thus each location carries a different energy than another. Remember to approach the devas with respect and love in your heart, and they will respond in kind.

Rock Water, or Natural Spring Water

This is one of the first environmental essences of the modern era, and it was made by Dr. Edward Bach. Instead of his usual flower remedies, he used a spring near his home, reasoning that the energy of the water carving through the rocks could also help his patients to flow more naturally and easily with the process of healing, the business of living. Said Dr. Bach, this essence will benefit "those who are very strict in their way of living; they deny themselves many of the joys and pleasures of life because they consider it might interfere with their work. They are hard masters to themselves. They wish to be well and strong and active, and will do anything which they believe will keep them so. They hope to be examples which will appeal to others who may then follow their ideas and be better as a result."

Natural springs which flow through rocks bring the energies of the deep earth, the flowing rains, winds and life-giving waters all together in one source. Essences made from natural artisanal springs are grounding and energizing. They allow us to be secure in ourselves and thus enjoy the flow of life more easily. Bach's favored sources of rock water were natural, holy springs known for their healing qualities. There are places like this in almost every town or county in the world – search your local folklore for such stories, or use your intuition and follow your heart. Healing waters are easy to identify by the lush quality of plant life and natural quiet around them, the peaceful yet invigorating effect they tend to have upon humans, and the reverence they encourage. Before you take rock water, always be sure to ask the spring's permission – there are generally powerful nature devas at work here.

Hot Springs

Another healing essence derives from an altogether different sort of spring. The warm waters of a hot spring augment the fire energies within us and are beneficial to those who feel alone in a big, cold world. They are nurturing, while also carrying the same grounding and strengthening energies of the other spring waters. It accesses the womb-like vibration of Mother Earth, enabling rebirth and soul renewal. It helps us save ourselves, become who we yearn to be, and see that we carry the seed of all possibilities within us.

Rivers and Streams

River essences are immensely helpful when we are feeling stuck or unable to move forward. The larger the body of water, the more it will work on "the big picture" – soul issues, life purpose, long-term illness. The smaller streams are good for working through specific issues such as work, relationship troubles, and acute illness. Keep in mind the natural flow of the water for your purposes. Does it flow quickly? Gently? Is it a wide, deep river like the Mississippi, or does it flow shallow over many rocks and boulders? Are the rocks in its basin quartz, linghams, granite? Is it inhabited by trout, otters, ducks, hippos, eels? Take into account everything you can about its habitat and character – sometimes working with these additional aspects of the river can also be helpful.

Oceans

The push and pull. The advance and retreat. A major influential aspect of the oceans is their tides. Much like working with the seasons, working with the oceans helps us to become one with the flow of time, to be easy with change and new developments. Life is a circle, and ocean energy can help you see things to completion, through to their next level. Another wonderful thing about the ocean is that it gets us in touch with our physical roots at a cellular level. Seawater contains, on average, around 85 minerals and its salinity is identical to amniotic fluid. Clearly, one cannot easily make an essence of amniotic fluid. When one is in need of birthing a new creation, an essence made from the ocean waves is just the thing.

Waterfalls

Waterfalls, be they large or small, are some of the most powerful phenomenon in the world. Their force can be used to create electrical power or to change the shape of the earth. Wanting to be swept away, swept up, and carried along in a torrent of joyful change? Waterfalls are a wonderful tool. They awaken the senses and invigorate the soul. Harness their vibration to combat anxiety, insomnia, and depression on an energetic level. Many people report feeling remarkably relaxed or sensual after being near at a waterfall. Scientists speculate this effect occurs because all waterfalls generate thousands of negative ions in the air, which in turn neutralizes positive ions in the air, which then enters your body and increases serotonin levels in the brain.

Glaciers

Patience, sir. Patience. The world wasn't made in a day. Take the beautiful rolling hills and small mountains of New England. My earth science teacher in seventh grade used to take pleasure in the fact these small hills were the wise old mountains of the United States. By contrast, the grandiose mountains of the West are young upstarts, untried and unmolded by glaciers or time. Ah, but the mountains of the East. They were groomed and shaped by millennia under the weight and grind of miles of ice, the glaciers of old. Rocks larger than houses were broken down, moved here and there, pushed to and fro.

Glaciers mix layers of earth into new configurations, plant seeds in locations previously unknown to their floral forefathers, and create new potentized ley lines. Glaciers give Mother Earth a moment to relax. They are like a spa treatment for the land. Tap into their energy with a glacial essence and receive the gift of patience, the quiet blessing of surrender and release, the ability to sit back and let "all good things come to those who wait." Learn the art of allowing, where we receive everything we want just by being who we really are. When it is time to grow and to move, we grow and we move. When it is time to melt and recede, we flow and we accede to a higher power, to Source, to all that is. Glaciers help us to see the big picture by acknowledging that we ARE the big picture. We are everything, and everything is part of us.

Mountains

Immoveable yet not inert. Mountains are often described as old men, wise and knowing. High in the clouds, they see all. Reaching into the sky, they are nearest the sun, the moon and the stars. Nearest, it often seems, to heaven, God and all the angels above.

Mountains have indeed stood the test of time, and they are wonderful sources of empowerment and strength. Some mountains were used for centuries as lookout posts – these mountains carry the energies of warriors and protections. Some mountains are extremely difficult to climb due to their inclines or their climate – such mountains imbue essences with the daring energies of adventurers and innovators, of success in the face of adversity. Some mountains are easy, quiet, serene. They will give your essence a sense of confidence and self-comfort.

Volcanoes

Volcanoes look like mountains, but they carry more of the feminine energy of the earth, more of the dark side of the crone. Volcanoes carry both the powers of destruction and rebirth within them. Their eruptions can kill and eradicate entire forests and wipe out life near and far, but their ash also has the ability to create rich new soil and wondrous ecosystems. Often they are associated with a particular local deity. And, more often than not this deity was considered a mother, a healer, and a woman not to be scorned or ignored, lest she unleash her wrath upon you. Capture the essence of a volcano in your bottle, and you will have at your fingers the power nothing less than the pure creative potential of the Earth herself. Volcanic essences can be helpful to those seeking justice (just make sure you are walking a path of truth) and needing to get in touch with the element of fire.

Ley Lines, Holy Places & Places of Power

You can tap into some particularly strong earth energy when you make an essence on a natural ley line or place of power. Ley lines are "the gridwork of the earth [which] runs everywhere in fine, electric blue lines, and some of these lines are stronger, wider, more turned on and tapped into by you humans. These are the places where humans have learned how to connect to the powers of Source…where time and space can cease to exist and you may become one with ALL THAT IS, in the blink of an eye." Ley lines are the energetic meridian channels of the planet. While veins and nerves run everywhere, as in the human body, some are stronger and more vital. These most powerful lines are those which most people refer to when they speak of ley lines. It has been found that many holy sites and places of power or healing line up when one uses a ruler across the globe. Even between many of the small towns in my area of New England, churches can be connected by straight lines. Local ley lines can be found through dowsing methods or maps, but often one only has to look for the places of legend, the holy sites.

When you do use a holy site for an essence, you are capturing not only the natural vibration of a empowered earth outlet, but also the centuries or millennia of prayer and healing magick that has further raised the power of the location. Remember – every sound ever generated goes on forever in its wave form. It never ceases to exist. Prayers are repeated throughout time, building upon one another and creating a never-ending crescendo of creation and intent. (Bear this is mind, too, when you send ill words out into the ether. They can never be taken back, and their vibration will exist for ever.)

The Auroras

Ah, the enchantment of the aurora borealis and aurora australis. If you ever have the chance to see an auroral event, know that you are experiencing something very, very special. These amazing lights in the night sky are created by the impact of energetically-charged solar particles upon as they collide with atoms in our atmosphere. It is literally an explosion of light energy. Many cultures believe that the lights are associated with Source energy, the Cree calling them a "Dance of Spirits" and the Germans, "Heaven Light."

Essences made under the light of an Aurora connect you to this heavenly dance. It is a connection to solar energies, and thus to the blueprint of our solar system and our planetary ascension plan. Clear karmic debris from your vibration and re-align with your true soul purpose.

Astrological Events

There are literally endless numbers of astrological alignments and conjunctions that you can harness for your own development. Work with Mercury Retrograde to better understand what is holding you back in your communications. Try Jupiter in Libra to encourage cooperation in the workplace or become more comfortable in social situations. If you wish to use the power of the stars and planets to make your essences, I recommend becoming familiar the impact of current astrological events. One of my favorite online resources is www.aquariuspapers.com.

Full Moons

The moon is associated with the divine feminine, with fertility and growth. Many of the most revered goddesses are connected with moon power, and their energy can be invoked through a full moon essence.

Energetically, when the moon is full, there is a sense of completion and celebration. Many believe that this is the most powerful, magical time of the month. If there is something you want to achieve, the full moon is the perfect time to state your intentions and focus your will on whatever it is you wish to accomplish. Make your essence, and then use it to set your plans in motion and bring your body into alignment with your soul.

Each full moon connects with a different astrological sign as well as its own season, so this, too can affect your essence. A full moon in Sagittarius will help you in academic pursuits or begin new projects; while a full moon in Virgo can help you get organized and pay more attention to detail. Generally, you will want to set your essence in the light of the moon for the three days before and the 1 day of the moon at it's fullest in order to capture its full energy.

New Moons

New moon energy is quite different from full moon energy. Now the night is at its darkest. You can see the stars at their best, but all else is obscured, hidden. It is a time that man, unable to see well in the dark, has conventionally been feared and associated with dark magic and secret knowledge. Of course, we know now that there is nothing to fear in the darkness. It is a time of renewal and rebirth, a time to end old patterns and disconnect from negativity. Essences made during the New Moon support us when we are trying to break old habits or get rid of unwanted energies. The best way to make a new moon essence is to set out your bowl of water on several days before the new moon and leave it out through the night of the new moon, so you can capture the cycle of diminishment through to its end.

Eclipses

There are two sorts of eclipses to experience on our planet: lunar and solar. Since we've been talking about the moon, let us first focus on what happens when this enters eclipse.

A lunar eclipse can only happen when the moon is full. As it passes behind the earth, for a few moments the full light of the sun can no longer illuminate it, and it takes on a beautiful reddish glow. Depending on the exact geometry of its position, the moon moves through its entire cycle in minutes or hours, going from full, to waning, to new, to waxing and full again. Thus a lunar eclipse is an especially powerful time to combine magical intentions of diminishment and creation. Perhaps you have a new business venture you want to try, but you need to release your fear of failure before you can succeed. Or maybe you are ready to find love, but first you must clear your internal blocks of distrust. Lunar eclipses empower you with earth energies so that you can move past your fears and bloom.

Solar eclipses, conversely, may only happen during a new moon. In a short time, the moon passes between the earth and the sun, obscuring the sun from our sight and creating darkness in the sky. Much as a lunar eclipse represents a miniature lunar month, a solar eclipse takes us through a mini-year – from full solar power, to waning, to the eclipse which may be equated with the winter equinox, to waxing, and back to full solar power, or summer equinox. So here we have the perfect moment to create an essence that will empower us through the year and enable us to move past any long-standing blockages or patterns.

Days of Power – Births, Deaths, New Years

As we've shown, essences can be made at any place or time. You can make an essence on any special day, whether it is a day acknowledged for it power by many or by one. An essence made on the day of a child's birth can be used later in life to return the subject to its original intention and physical blueprint. An essence made at a death can help us to accept the completion of the journey, to celebrate the reconnection of soul with source. Make an essence to gather the vibration of Fire Dog at the Chinese New Year, or encourage victory and liberty on Bastille Day in France. Make an essence at 11:11 to connect with the high-vibration guides who are helping humanity along to its higher evolution.

Choose your time. Choose your place. Set out your water in its bowl or glass, and let the magic that surrounds you, the blessings of the earth imbue your essence with the healing power you choose.

Incorporating Homeopathy

Homeopathy is quantum vibrational medicine. It began in 1790 with the studies of Dr. Samuel Hahnemann, and his belief that like could cures like. One of his first personal confirmations of this idea was his research into cinchona bark, a South American tree bark that was being used to treat malarial symptoms. Malaria free himself, he noted that the ingestion of cinchona by a healthy person would produce malarial symptoms. Encouraged by this pronounced case of like curing like, Hahnemann delved further into his research and soon had developed an entire system of medicine. His students continued the studies and founded schools in the United States in the 1800s, and homeopathy experienced widespread support in Europe and India during the 1900s. These days, homeopathic remedies are sold in most pharmacies throughout Europe, and have been proven in many studies to have a pronounce effect that is verifiably stronger than a placebo medicine.

So how does it work?

Homeopathic practitioners use minute, molecularly diluted doses of something that produces the same symptoms to alleviate a particular condition: for example, if you are suffering from an allergic reaction, you might take remedy of histaminum or apis millefica (histamine or bee venom). Don't be afraid – the remedy you are taking has been diluted with water anywhere from 3 to 1000 times, so much so that there is **no measurable molecular evidence or trace remaining** of the original extract.

Homeopathic remedies begin their life as full-strength "mother" tinctures, the same sort of tincture an herbalist would traditionally use. It is then transformed into a homeopathic dilution by placing one drop of mother tincture in 100 drops of solution, followed by a shaking of the bottle. Homeopathic remedies come in many dosages, the most common being 6x, 30c, 200c and 1m, ranging from low to high doses respectively. The numbers indicate how many times the remedy has been diluted. So a 6x has repeated the dilution process six times.

The part that really drives most modern scientists crazy? The more diluted the remedy, the stronger it is believed to be.

Intention, in vibrational remedies, is everything. Each time the remedy is diluted and activated through the shaken, the remedy is potentized. Weaker dosages are generally used for acute situations and can be taken as often as every 10-15 minutes. High potencies (such as 200c and 1m) address chronic vibrational imbalances and are generally used at monthly or weekly intervals. There is more information about potencies and how to create your own remedies in the following chapter.

Now, remember, you are an energetic being. In the theory of homeopathy, you are having a negative reaction to the sting of an insect because vibrationally there is something in you that does not resonate with the energy of the sting. Your vibration needs to be finely tuned and brought into alignment. When you align with the vibration of a sting or an allergic reaction at a quantum, homeopathic level with purposeful intention, you are energetically signaling your body that you would like to come into alignment with that energy.

Homeopathy is very useful as an adjunct to both allopathic and other alternative therapies. Many allopathic doctors in the United States are taking cues from their overseas peers and are beginning to suggest basic homeopathic remedies to their patients. Arnica, in particular, is enjoying great popularity among both physical therapists and surgeons. Studies have shown that not only will Arnica decrease muscle pain, but it seems to speed healing and improve recovery times after operations if taken during the days before and after surgery.

For many people, cell salts are an easy way to begin their first foray into homeopathy. There are 12 cell salts which are present in everyone's body. When any of these cell salts is deficient (which often happens these days due to poor nutrition and depleted farm soils) the tissues and organs of the body begin to deteriorate and function poorly. Low homeopathic dilutions of cell salts return the salts to the body in minute dosages so that the body can regain balance. 6x dilutions are generally considered optimal for restoring harmony to the body.

If you delve into homeopathy for any period of time, chances are you will stumble upon the theory of miasms. The word miasm was chosen by Hahnemann in 1828 for his text, The Chronic Diseases, to describe the idea of underlying infections in the body, infectious "fogs" we are all born with, imprinted upon our DNA from generations past and clouding our otherwise perfect bodies. Further miasmic contamination is possible through human contact and vaccinations, too. Hahnemann posited that all current illnesses and dis-eases begin with the weakening effect that these miasms have upon our systems. If a person is seriously interested in eradicating all dis-ease from the body, further investigation into the miasms is strongly recommended by most homeopaths.

The first three miasms Hahnemann introduced, and still considered the most prevalent, are Psora, Syphilitic and Sycosis. Psora dis-eases include most chronic illnesses and dysfunctions of the body and are believed to produce 85% of all illnesses, especially those relating to skin problems. Its chief remedies include Sulphur, Zinc, Silicea, Calc Carb, Nat Mur, Causticum and Lycopodium. Syphilitic miasms derive from ancient venereal diseases and are characterized by blood and skeletal issues, and a wide range of psychological dis-orders. The primary remedies are Lycopodium, Phosphorus, Arsenicum and Mercury. Sycosis derives from Gonorrhea and affects many current STDs, warts, joints, mucous production and urination. Main remedies include Thuja, Sepia, Causticum, Kali sulph and Nat Sulph.

Over a hundred single remedies are available at most local health food stores, as well as through mail order online. Many regular supermarkets and pharmacies are also beginning to carry homeopathic combination remedies in the cold and flu aisle, especially now that the FDA has banned over-the-counter cold remedies for children.

Some of the best companies on the market are Boiron, NatraBio, Hylands, Walsh, and Metagenics. Remedies generally come in the form of small sugar pills or liquid alcohol or glycerin bases. Single remedies are good for specific conditions, while combination formulas are great if you don't know exactly what the cause of the condition is, because they will treat a multitude of symptoms and causes.

The advice of an experienced homeopathic doctor can be invaluable – most have a strict comprehensive diagnostic routine which they follow. A good website to start with, if you are interested in more information about homeopathy, is www.abchomeopathy.com.

Common Homeopathic Remedies

Aconitum Napellus is most recommended for panic attacks, fear and anxiety. It is also used at the initial onset of a cold to shorten the duration of illness and to reduce fevers.

Allium Cepa is used for watery coughs, runny noses and eyes, and hay fever.

Apis Mellifica is used to counteract allergic reactions that involve swelling, especially insect bites.

Argentum Nitricum is helpful in cases of stage fright or nervousness. It is also used to reduce body tremors and balance issues.

Arnica Montana can be taken either internally for generalized trauma or pain, or used topically as a gel or cream to ease bruising and muscle injuries. As mentioned previously, it is believed to hasten healing and reduce discomfort after surgical procedures.

Arsenicum Album is touted to fight food poisoning, fevers and reduce vomiting. It is also used to reduce burning and throbbing headaches, sore throats and painful eczema conditions.

Belladonna is used to combat fevers, colds and sinusitis. It is relaxing to the body, useful when there has been trauma or shock, and may improve sleep conditions.

Bioplasma is a combination formula that includes all 12 of the single cell salt remedies for easy optimization and harmonizing of tissue functions in the body.

Bryonia Alba helps reduce nausea and digestive troubles and is also used to improve muscle and joint pain.

Calcarea Carbonica is used to benefit tooth health and cradle cap.

Calcarea Fluorica is a cell used to maintain healthy skin and teeth. Raw, rough skin, spider veins or tooth decay may be symptoms of Cal Fluor deficiency, as may low self-esteem. Cal Fluor is often used as an alternative to Fluoride supplements and treatments. It also benefits muscle sprains.

Calcarea Phosphorica is a cell salt that promotes bone health and growth. If one has is feeling weak or unmotivated, or has growing pains, aches or bone problems then one may be deficient in Cal Phos.

Calcarea Sulphurica is a cell salt whose deficiency symptoms tend to manifest in weakened immunity and soft tissues. This means that injuries might heal quite slowly and one might be prone to infections and lymph issues. Emotionally, one may present with depression, laziness or apathy.

Causticum is used in both children and adults to decrease bed-wetting and incontinence.

Chamomilla is perfect for young children who are teething or restless. Use it to help calm anyone who is prone to stress or snappish. It is also indicated for inflammation and fever.

Cimicifuga Racemosa helps reduce upper back pain and relaxes the uterus to combat painful menstruation.

Cinchona Officinalis fights bloating and helps stop diarrhea.

Coffea Cruda is used to combat insomnia, relaxing the mind so that sleep may occur.

Ferrum Phosphate helps the oxygen delivery system of the body, and helps invigorate the senses. It is also helpful for inflammation and immunity.

Graphites reduces scarring and helps skin heal itself.

Hepar Sulphuris Calcareum is used to improve hoarse, dry coughs and sore throats.

Histaminum Hydrochloricum is used to lessen allergic responses caused by over-stimulated immune systems.

Hypericum Perforatum is a must have for any first aid kit, and is used for nerve injuries and shooting pains. Keep on hand for accidents, puncture wounds, and spinal injuries. Hypericum is also used for depression.

Ignatia Amara is used to combat everyday stress and tension, and is very helpful for those who feel over sensitized to mundane drama or conflict.

Kali Carbonicum is generally recommended for relieving soreness and strengthening the lower back.

Kali Muriaticum is a cell salt that governs vitality and well-being in the body. If one is deficient in this salt they may often be sick, tired or suffer from inflammation in the body. It is a good remedy for colds with nasal congestion.

Kali Phosphoricum is another cell salt ruling the body's ability to adapt and process energy. Deficiencies tend to present with emotional and physical exhaustion following times of stress and irritability. Used for migraines and tension headaches.

Kali Sulphuricum is a cell salt ruling the production and processing of oils of the body. Lack of both mental and physical fluidity are symptoms of Kali Sulph imbalances, including dry or oily skin, digestive problems, and anxiety. Often used to combat colds that are settled into the sinuses and characterized by thick yellow mucous.

Lachesis Mutus is used for hormonal imbalances and menopausal symptoms, especially hot flashes.

Ledum Palustre has been used traditionally to heal insect bites. In recent years, it has been used in various clinical trials to treat Lyme disease with good results. Stephen Tobin, DVM, recommends "one pellet of Ledum 1M three times a day for three days. I have been using Borrellia burgdorferi 60X nosode, a homeopathic preparation, as a preventative for Lyme disease in dogs. I give orally one dose daily for one week, then one dose a week for one month, then one dose every six months. One homeopathic MD runs titers on all his [human] Lyme disease patients, both before and after treatment with Ledum, and has found that there is a constant decline in titer after Ledum."

Lycopodium Clavatum is generally used to decrease abdominal bloating and gas. It is also recommended to remove aluminum from the body and combat the Tubercular miasm.

Magnesium Phosphorica is a cell salt that works with the muscles and nervous system. It is often recommended for abdominal cramping, particularly during menstruation. Use with ferrum phosphate to fight general muscle cramping or inflammation.

Natrum Muriaticum is the first of the sodium cell salts and helps to regulate water and fluids in the body. When is one deficient in Nat Mur, one might experience bloating, headaches and suffer from excess mucous. Try using it during allergy season to reduce runny noses.

Natrum Phosphoricum is another cell salt and regulates digestion. It is often indicated in cases of acid reflux or heartburn.

Natrum Sulphuricum is a cell salt involved in pancreatic function. It is used to improve lung issues that are worsened by dampness.

Nux Vomica helps control nausea, heartburn, vomiting and diarrhea, making it useful for both illnesses and motion sickness.

Pulsatilla Nigricans is good for colds and infections with thick, yellow discharge. Associated with any ailments involving swelling, it is used especially for bruises and swollen joints.

Rhus Toxicodendron is used by many people to improve arthritic conditions and loosen their joints. Rhus tox is also helpful during the initial stages of poison ivy reactions, to shorten or lessen the condition.

Ruta Graveolens is used to decrease eye strain, glaucoma and frontal headaches, especially those deriving from poor lighting or computer usage.

Sepia helps to stabilize the moods and is used by many to combat depression, bipolar tendencies and gynecological troubles.

Silicea is a cell salt that helps regulates perspiration and is necessary for the healthy growth of nails, hair and skin. It is often recommended in cases of overwork, when demands become overwhelming or stressful and the mind or body begin to suffer from fatigue.

Sulphur improves colitis, digestion, acne and skin rashes. It has also been used to diminish cellulite and menopausal symptoms. In men, it may help reproductive issues, and in children it is often recommended to discourage temper tantrums and sleep aversion.

Thuja Occidentalis is used both topically and internally to get rid of warts and combat the herpes virus and venereal miasms. It is also good for mood and sleep disorders.

Making your own homeopathic remedies

Homeopathic remedies are widely available on the internet, from homeopathic practitioners and doctors, and at many health food markets and pharmacies. It is always best to use homeopathics under the supervision of a trained professional, and the manufacturing process of remedies on the market are strictly monitored and regulated. However, sometimes one does not have access to the remedies they need, whether due to location, cost or rarity. In such cases, it is rather simple to make one's own remedy at home.

First, you need the item you are making your remedy from. If you are allergic to the air around you, you can collect its offending pollutants by leaving a bowl of pure distilled water out on a table for several hours. More commonly, you will want to make your homeopathic base or mother by infusing the item into a jar or bottle filled with a 50/50 water/alcohol solution for at least several days. Ideally, pulverize, macerate or powder the item first. If you are having autoimmune issues, you might use your own hair or fingernail. If a medicine or food is causing an issue, crush and add it to the jar. You can also use mother flower essences or herbal tinctures as the base for your homeopathic remedy.

What you will need:

- A glass jar with a non-reactive lid

- A base for your remedy

- Pure distilled water

First, you need to decide what potency you wish to produce. The numeral in a potency denotes how many times the remedy has been diluted and then succused. The letter after the numeral indicates the amount of dilution at each step before succusion and follows the roman numeral system. So a 6X remedy has gone through both steps, dilution at a 1:9 ratio and succusion, six times. A 6C remedy has been diluted at a 1:99 ratio and succussed six times. M remedies are diluted at a 1:1000 ratio and succussed. The more times a remedy has gone through the steps of dilution and succusion, the more potent it is. X remedies tend to address acute, short-term situations while M remedies generally address miasmic, underlying tendencies on an energetic level. C remedies fall somewhere in between the two.

Say you want to make a 12X potency. Fill your mason jar about halfway with 9 parts water and 1 part remedy base. You can use spring water or distilled water, although distilled water will contain the fewest contaminants and trace minerals which could potentially interact with your remedy. Put the lid on your jar, and succuss the remedy. What does this mean? Succussing is the method used to potentized remedies, or activate their vibrational patterns, and may be done in a variety of ways. Some homeopaths prefer to hold the jar in one hand and gently pound the jar into their other palm 30-50 times. Other homeopaths vigorously shake the remedy for 60 seconds and then gently slam the jar on their palm or a book on a desk three times. Repeat these steps 11 more times, diluting and succussing each time, and you will have your very own homemade 12X remedy. These water based remedies should be stored in the refrigerator and consumed within 12-14 days. If you wish your remedy to have a longer shelf life, use alcohol or glycerin with water in your final dilution (you want the final solution to have 25% grain alcohol, 50% brandy or vodka, or 50% glycerin, with the remainder being water including your potency)

One way I love to work with homeopathic remedies is to relieve chronic allergies. I begin with a low potency formula which combines the allergen culprits in homeopathic form, as well as histaminum, all at 6X. Formulas like this can be found at most health stores for under $15. I take the formula by the dropperfull every 10-30 minutes whenever I suffer from the allergy. Then, when I get down to the last dropper of the bottle, instead of buying a second bottle, I **make a stronger potency bottle** by refilling the bottle with water, adding this last dropper to the bottle and succussing it. Then I keep taking the remedy as usual. Within several weeks I am at a much higher potency and working on a different energetic level of my being. The longer you do this, the more levels of your being you are hitting, thereby addressing the dis-ease in more aspects – emotionally, spiritually, physically. I tried this for the first time 7 years ago, virtually curing myself of spring tree pollen allergies, and have many friends and clients who have benefitted from the same protocol. Some years the allergy will recur in mild form – I begin the protocol again and generally am cleared of the allergy within a few days. This is a wonderful thing, since spring is my favorite season!

Electro-Magnetic Quantum Healing Technologies

In this chapter we have perhaps the most complex of the vibrational medicines, technologies which address the integrity of the bio-field using electrical frequencies and feedback. These therapies all use machines to measure or adjust electrical impulses in the body to remedy dis-ease.

Biofeedback & Kinesiology

The term biofeedback encompasses a wide range of screening and therapy devices used these days which monitor the body's reactions to outside stimuli by measuring body temperature, electrical conductivity, muscle strength and brainwaves. For most practitioners what comes to mind when they hear the word "biofeedback" are technologies which find their roots in the research of Dr. Reinhardt Voll. Measuring electrical conductivity of the skin in the 1940's, Dr. Voll discovered that all acupuncture points exhibit measurably higher conductivity than the rest of the body. Upon further testing, he found that when the Qi flow of meridian is compromised, points on that system will show lower readings, too. Liver disease will manifest in poor readings in points which relate to that organ; even more interesting, just holding a vial of purgative medicine would lower conductivity in stomach acupoints. Out of this discovery Dr. Voll developed the theory of **Electro-Acupuncture** (EAV), whereby one could asses acupuncture points using energetic assessment technology. This technology is also called **Electro-Dermal Screening** (EDS) or **Meridian Stress Assessment** (MSA). These conductivity meters are used to indirectly measure the Qi flow at specific points, which in turn indicates the health of the organ to which the point refers.

Biofeedback may be a helpful tool to any health practitioner in diagnosing impaired function in the body. Most frequently, however, a client might see biofeedback being used to determine which remedy will work best for them. Various remedies can be tested and measured along with the patient's own readings to indicate which bottle might improve or hinder Qi flow. Neutral or negative (50 or less) readings suggest a poor effect on the body, while positive readings (50+) indicate that the client would benefit from a particular remedy. Diet and allergy response can be tested in a similar manner, without the client ever actually being exposed to any substances.

A more primitive, but very effective form of biofeedback is **kinesiology** or muscle testing. This form of biofeedback uses the body's own physical response to a substance be your guide. The idea here is that the body's bio-field will either be weakened or strengthened by any substance that it comes in contact with. Testing vials containing dilutions of various fungi or viruses may be tested to show the presence of that dis-ease in the body, or a bottle of pills might be held to see what its effect would be. Muscle testing is best done in pairs, with the testee's eyes closed so that they do not know which remedies or vials they are holding. In this case, but it can also be done by oneself.

Muscle testing is very easy and there is no need for a computer or technology. When working in pairs, first a baseline must be established. Have the testee stand or sit comfortably and close their eyes. Now ask the testee to put their non-dominant arm out straight to side. Press firmly upon the arm to determine a baseline reaction while the testee tries to keep their arm parallel with the ground. Now have the testee hold a bottle, still with eyes closed, and repeat the test. Was it easier to push down their arm? The easier it is, the more the testee's biofield has been weakened by the substance, and the less good it will do in their body.

To conduct muscle testing on yourself without a partner, try one of the following methods. The first method requires the use of both your hands. Place the substance in your lap and form a circle with your left thumb and forefinger. Now press your right thumb and forefinger together, and place them within the O made by your other hand's fingers. Try to use them as a vise to force open the other fingers' circle by opening them within the O, while also trying to hold the outer circle closed. If you can easily open the outer circle, your body has been weakened by the substance and it is not good for you. Many people enjoy this first method, although I personally have had varying degrees of success with it and find it relatively unreliable. I prefer this second method. Stand up and hold the test substance in your dominant hand. Take a few deep breathes and center your mind, aligning with your soul self. Now close your eyes and hold the substance just in front of your forehead at the third eye. Slowly move your hand down your body to your solar plexus. If your body leans towards your hand as it moves, it will benefit your biofield. If your body leans backwards, away from the substance, then it will not benefit you at this time.

Bioenergetic Medicine

Many people are introduced to biofeedback techniques when they first start on the vibrational healing path. Eventually, this naturally leads one to the field of **Bioenergetics**. These remedies are believed to carry the energy frequencies to destroy infectious agents and boost healing in the body.

As discovered by Dr. Voll, the electromagnetic frequency of bodily tissue changes when the body is unwell. At first, the stressed tissue will produce feelings of fatigue, soreness, and a weakened immune system. Eventually, the body itself will begin to decline, manifesting physical or mental symptoms of dis-ease, even cancer.

Bioenergetic medicine uses an electromagnetic charging plate to imbue a natural substance (generally water) with the frequencies that will destroy a particular organism or virus. Dr. Royal Raymond Rife discovered that specific electrical frequencies could be used to target and destroy harmful bacteria while leaving other cells unharmed. This same idea is used to make bioenergetic remedies. They are taken in a similar fashion to homeopathic medicines and, like homeopathics, are particularly well suited to the treatment of miasms and other underlying agents of dis-ease. Pollutants and heavy metals may be addressed, too.

Most remedies can be ordered in the form of dosage bottles which are taken 1-3 times daily for a prescribed course of time. Three good sources are David Alan Slater's international organization, www.healerswhoshare.com, Ergopathic Resources at www.ergopathics.com, and the makers of Al-Khemi Antidotes at www.earthmotherherbs.org.

Frequency Generators

Bioresonance is a term used to describe the interaction between your body and external frequencies. There are many vibrational therapies which fall under the category of bioresonance. Italian Scientist Pier Luigi Ighina showed in his experiments that damaged or diseased cells can be healed by exposure to a magnetic field oscillator generating the vibratory rate of healthy cells. This idea has strong roots in real science and many machines exist today on the market that work on within this basic premise. Some are reliable, while others remain unproven in scientific trials. One of the most reputable and widely accepted forms of bioresonant therapies is the frequency generator, often called a Rife machine after the work of Royal Rife.

Rife machines emit a wide range of electric frequencies through hand-held rods or foot-plates. The body receives a low electrical current on a specified frequency. One might feel a slight tingling in the hands or feet, or nothing at all. Generally, it is described as a pleasant sensation, if anything is felt.

Each frequency is believed to address a particular ailment, with different frequencies referred for specific viruses, bacteria and even cancers. Using inversion techniques, frequency therapies are also recommended for the detoxification of heavy metals and other contaminants in the body.

There are large, open libraries available online, where users in the Rife communities are constantly adding their own experiential feedback and results. Some findings are quite clinical and scientific in nature, while others are more personal and perhaps biased. Dr. Hulda Clark contributed a large amount of research to this field in the 1990s, identifying specific frequencies which affect various bacteria. Frequency generators have been shown in numerous studies to produce positive results, and are used extensively in health clinics throughout Eastern Europe and Russia. Rife machines are easy to use, one simply sets them to the prescribed set of frequencies and holds the bars for 1-10 minutes per frequency (some sets may have up to 20 frequencies in them, so treatment generally takes about 20-30 minutes). There are also frequencies which have been determined to jumpstart the immune system and help improve the body's overall ability to heal itself. Sets are repeated over the course of several days, or even weeks in the case of chronic disease.

I have used frequency generators, both on their own and in conjunction with other vibrational healing methods. I find them to be quite helpful, especially when used with homeopathy or flower essences, and have personally felt results in detoxification processes, flu treatments, and intra-muscular pain relief. The machine itself is not cheap, generally costing at least a few hundred dollars, however if you have easy access to one I do recommend giving it a try as a conjunctive therapy.

Should you decide to purchase a frequency generator for yourself, invest in one that will allow you to program whatever frequencies you desire and support ranges from 0.1Hertz to 20,000 Hertz. Machines that further allow you to pre-program and run an entire set of frequencies may be worth the extra expense, since they may save you quite a bit of time and work, especially if you are planning to use the machine every day.

You Are the Charging Plate

If you have made it this far through my book, then you have probably noticed that I hold three basic beliefs:

1. Intention is everything.

2. You are an energetic being.

3. All energy is connected.

So how do these beliefs fit together in the context of vibrational healing? It's quite simple, really. When you get down to it, physical medicines or bio-energetically charged vials are not required to heal your body. You don't need a charging plate to make medicine, and you don't need a Rife machine to blast bacterial particulates apart. You are the charging plate. You are the Rife machine. You are an energetic being, a quantum construction living in a realm of pure energy, and you don't really need these things. Although they can and will help, you do not need them.

Quantum mechanics has proven that all particles are essentially pure energy with no tangible matter. The closer science looks at matter, the more they find that there is nothing there. At an atomic level, we are empty space. When you look closely at an atom it is literally 99.9999999999999% empty space. The rest? It is a nucleon, which is also 99.999% space made up of quarks. These quarks, too, are 99.999% space. Where does it end? It doesn't.

We are space. And we are energy. Our bodies contain enough energy on an atomic level to provide power to .1% of the entire world's population.

We are simply holograms, energetic constructs operating in a theatre of divine creation. Our energy flows through space as waves and particles, interacting with other waves and particles to create the response that we are expecting.

Physics has shown, time and again, that matter behaves as we expect it to. When we watch an experiment, whether "we" are human eyes and ears or simply a mechanical recording device, we alter the behavior of the particles that comprise our physical reality. If we want a photon to behave as a particle, it will. But if we want it to behave as a wave, it will do that, too. Which is it? Which are we? Physical being or spirit and energy?

The simple answer? We're both.

So let's take that a step further, and bring it back into the context of healing. You want to work with a particular homeopathic remedy so that you can alter your biofield in a specific way. Unfortunately, you car is in the shop and you can't get to the store for a few days. You want the remedy now. What can you do?

Become the charging plate.

Make your own homeopathic remedy, simply by placing a glass of water on a piece of paper with the name of the remedy. Intend to connect your water with the energy of the remedy. When you feel the water has been properly charged, take the water the way you would take the remedy.

Or don't even make the remedy. Simply intend to connect with the remedy in whatever way best suits you. Find a picture of the remedy online and place your hand on the computer screen, aligning with the remedy until you feel you've accomplished your goal. Or print the name on a piece of paper and align with the words. Or visualize yourself having the vial, opening the vial, and ingesting the remedy.

Sound too strange? We've all heard of the placebo effect. Science would like us to feel that the placebo effect is a bad thing. That people believing something works, and then having it work, is undesirable. Science acts like because the sugar pill was simply a sugar pill, this should negate the **important fact that taking the sugar pill created a measurable improvement in the physical and emotional condition of the believer.** Unfortunately for Big Pharma, over the last couple decades the placebo response seems to be getting stronger, making it more difficult for new drugs to pass FDA trials – placebos are starting to rank just as well as many new drugs. Even old drugs, like Prozac, are performing worse in trials against placebos. This is bad news for the shareholders in large pharmaceutical companies, but good news for proponents of vibrational medicine and those who study the biofield.

Personally, I find the placebo effect to be a desirable and significant occurrence. Let's look at it a bit more closely. What exactly is happening here? When a person consciously decides to ingest a physical medicine, and are not aware that they are ingesting a sugar pill, they are aligning with the energy of the physical medicine. If patients are treated more warmly by their physician, the effect rises another 20%. If a person is told that the drug will have bad side effects, these can occur, too. Placebo effects are also called "expectation effects," for this very reason. In general, placebo effects occur in 30-40% of a population, although some studies show rates indicating that nearly everyone experiences a placebo effect. In studies where patients were treated more warmly and with extra contact by their physician the placebo rate increased from 40% up to 60%. Perhaps this explains the fact that placebos works even better for animals and children, who have no real expectations but are generally treated with greater warmth and care than adults.

I have found in my own family that giving them remedies without their knowledge, such as placing a homeopathic in the water they take to school or work, will produce an effect that other people notice although no one has any idea that I've given my children or husband anything. So. Are the remedies actually working? Or does my entire community experience a placebo effect based on my intention and connection to the quantum web of energy? Does it even matter why they work? My son concentrates better at school since I added Clematis flower essence to his water bottle. My husband is happier and experiencing less pain with arnica and silicea homeopathics. Everyone benefits.

As the Course in Miracles says, "there is no order of miracles." Miracles are miracles, large or small. Healing is healing, large or small. Every aspect of your reality is an energetic construct, large or small. Every piece of physical matter is an amalgam of quantum energy aligning with intent. All you need to do is figure out the best way for you to work within this construct. For some people, flower essences might work best; for others, conventional medicine. For many, a combination of the two will speak to the division they have created between their physical body and their spirit, the better to heal the rift between the two and create a more harmonious situation in this reality. And for still others, the basic realization that they are the charging plate will create the slight shift in perspective they need to embark upon their path to personal healing and comfort.

The remedies in this book are instruments of healing. They are tools that help you fix your attention and intent so that you may better harmonize with the flow of energy around you. Just like a scalpel or a pill, the remedies are not the healing itself, nor are there any guarantees that they will always work.

If they don't work, does it mean that you didn't try hard enough, that you expected the wrong outcome or that you are wanting to be ill? Absolutely not. It simply means that a particular tool of healing is not right for you at this time, not aligned with your vibration or compatible with your current life-path. The actual healing itself may not be right for you at this time. Maybe there is a lesson to be learned. Or maybe your higher self, your oversoul, your infinite-I, is just wanting to have this experience of illness or discomfort. Don't worry. It will pass, as does everything. The one guarantee you have in this lifetime is that things will change.

Be open. Be joyful. Be ready for whatever comes your way, for there's always something coming, and it's all part of the grand design. Your design? Maybe. Maybe not. But you are here, so why not play the game and enjoy the ride?

INDEX

B

bacteria, 48
balance, 186
balancing, 63
barberry, 87
basil, 46
bay, 46
bed-wetting, 187
bee-balm, 87
beech, 87
begonia, 87
belladonna, 186
benzoin, 46
bergamot, 47
beta waves, 71
binaural beats, 73
bioenergetic medicine, 198
biofeedback, 195
biofield, 14
biophotonic therapy, 65
bioplasma, 186
bioresonance, 199
bipolar disorder, 137, 190
birth, 104
bites, 186
black, 23, 63, 156
black tourmaline, 142
black-eyed susan, 88
bladder, 24
blame, 106, 137
bleeding heart, 88
bloating, 187, 189
blockages, 28, 33, 35, 38, 106, 139,
    151, 160, 180
blood, 29, 44, 45, 61, 64, 65, 66, 68,
    88, 106, 119, 130, 132, 134, 143,
    144, 145, 151, 167, 184
blood brain barrier, 45
bloodroot, 88
bloodstone, 130
blue, 24, 25, 26, 59, 62, 148, 176
bluebell, 89

blueprint, 5, 20, 62, 91, 100, 150, 177,
    180
boji stones, 131
bones, 16, 58, 67, 74, 95, 112, 166,
    167
borage, 89
bougainvillea, 89
brain, 18, 44, 45, 70, 71, 72, 73, 74,
    93, 129, 140, 173, 233
brain waves, 70
brown, 23, 61
bruises, 49, 190
bryonia alba, 187
buddha, 135, 148
bull thistle, 89
burns, 49, 50, 67, 138
burr cucumber, 90
business, 139
butterbur, 90
buttercup, 90
butterfly bush, 91

C

caduceus, 19
calcarea carbonica, 187
calcarea fluorica, 187
calcarea phosphorica, 187
calcarea sulphurica, 187
calcite, 131
calm, 86, 118, 165
calming, 3, 29, 44, 46, 48, 49, 50, 51,
    54, 55, 61, 62, 89, 106, 121, 136,
    138, 145, 152, 165, 168
cancer, 45, 59, 64, 66, 67, 103, 162,
    198, 223, 224, 232
canna lily, 91
carnelian, 23, 132
causticum, 187
cedarwood, 47
celandine, 91
celestobarite, 132
cell salts, 183, 186, 187, 188, 189, 190
cellular renewal, 129

T

References & Resources

Altomonte RPh, C. Kampo: The Japanese Art of Herbal Healing. Accessed at www.ittendojo.org.

Azeemi, S. and Raza, S.M., "A Critical Analysis of Chromotherapy and Its Scientific Evolution", Evid Based Complement Alternat Med. 2005 December; 2(4): 481–488.

Bach Flower Essences, Articles and Biography of Dr. Edward Bach, Accessed at www.bachflower.com

"Basic Explanation Of The Electrodermal Screening Test And The Concepts Of Bio-Energetic Medicine", American Association of Acupuncture and Bio-Energetic Medicine, Accessed at www.healthy.net.

Begley, M. "The Five Elemental Chakras of Polarity Therapy", 2003

Begley, M. "The Negative Pole of the Fundamental Field", 2010.

Bellows, W. Floral Acupuncture: Applying the Flower Essences of Dr. Bach to Acupuncture Sites, Crossing Press, 2005.

Beston, H. Herbs and the Earth: An Evocative Excursion into the Lore & Legend of Our Common Herbs. David R. Godine, 1935.

Bird, C and Tompkins, P. The Secret Life of Plants, Harper & Row, 1973.

Brailing, B. Light Years Ahead : The Illustrated Guide to Full Spectrum and Colored Light in Mindbody Healing.

Brennan, B. Hands of Light : A Guide to Healing Through the Human Energy Field, NY: Bantam, 1988.

Capra, F. The Tao of Physics: An Exploration of the Parallels between Modern Physics and Eastern Mysticism, Shambhala, 2010.

Capra, F. The Web of Life: A New Scientific Understanding of Living Systems, Anchor, 1997.

Carper, J. Miracle Cures: Dramatic New Scientific Discoveries Revealing the Healing Powers of Herbs, Vitamins, and Other Natural Remedies. HarperCollins Publishers, 1997.

Castleman, M. Nature's Cures. Rodale Press, 1996.

Chen, Ph.D., M.P.H, K. "An Analytic Review of Studies on Measuring Effects of External Qi in China," Alternative Therapies. July/Aug 2004, VOL. 10. No.4.

Chitty RPP, RCST, John & Muller MEd, RPP, RCST, Maria Louise. Energy Exercises: Easy Exercises for Health and Vitality, New Leaf, 2002.

Chopra, D. Quantum Healing: Exploring the Frontiers of Mind/Body Medicine. Bantam, 1990.

Cointreau, M. Grounding and Clearing: Being Present in the New Age, Earth Lodge Publications, 2008

Cointreau, M. Natural Animal Healing: An Earth Lodge Guide to Pet Wellness, Earth Lodge Publications, 2006.

Cointreau, S. Energy Healing for Animals and Their Owners: An Earth Lodge Guide to Pet Wellness, Earth Lodge Publications, 2009.

Cohen, K. "What is Qigong?" Qigong Research and Practice Center. Accessed at http://www.qigonghealing.com/

Cram, Dr. J. "Five Clinical Studies Demonstrate the Effectiveness of Flower Essence Therapy in the Treatment of Depression", Calix: International Journal of Flower Essence Therapy, Volume 1, Flower Essence Society

Davis, S. Butterflies Are Free To Fly: A New and Radical Approach to Spiritual Evolution. L&G Productions LLC, 2010.

De Giorgio, Dr. L. "Color Therapy – Chromotherapy", 2000-2012, Accessed at www.deeptrancenow.com/colortherapy.htm

Dharmananda Ph.D., S. Kampo Medicine: The Practice of Chinese Herbal Medicine in Japan. Institute for Traditional Medicine, Portland, Oregon.

Dobelis, I.N., Editor. Magic and Medicine of Plants. Pleasantville, NY: The Reader's Digest Assoc, 1990.

Duke, J.A. & Foster, S. Peterson Field Guides: Eastern/Central Medicinal Plants, Boston: Houghton Mifflin Company, 1990.

EAV, The Basics, 2013, Meridian Energies, The Center for BioDynamic Studies. Accessed at www.meridianenergies.net.

Eden, Articles and Information, 2007-2012, Accessed at www.edenisnow.com.

EFT Technique Videos and Coaching, Boundless Living Challenge with Bob Doyle.

Emoto, M. The Hidden Messages in Water, 2005, Atria Books.

Enwemeka, PT, PhD, FACSM, C. "Therapeutic Light", Rehab Management: The Interdisciplinary Journal of Rehabilitation, Jan/Feb 2004. Accessed at http://www.rehabpub.com/features/1022004/2.asp

Firebrace, P. & Hill, S. Acupuncture: How It Works, How It Cures. Keats Publishing, 1994.

Fischer-Rizzi, S. The Complete Aromatherapy Handbook: Essential Oils for Radiant Health. Sterling, 1991.

Fleischman, Dr. G. Acupuncture: Everything You Ever Wanted to Know. Station Hill Openings, 1998.

Flower Essence Society Scientific Studies, Articles and Research, Accessed through membership at http://www.flowersociety.org/research.htm

Geddes, Dr. N & Lockie, Dr. A. The Complete Guide to Homeopathy the Principles & Practices of Treatment, Dorling-Kindersley, 1995.

Gordon, R. Quantum-Touch: The Power to Heal, North Atlantic, 2006.

Gray, P. The Organic Horse: The Natural Management of Horses Explained. David & Charles, 2001.

Green, M. & Keville, K. Aromatherapy: A Complete Guide to the Healing Art. The Crossing Press, 1995.

Grimes, W. "Vets and Physicians Find Research Parallels", New York Times, 09/10/2012.

Hall, J. The Crystal Bible Volumes 1 & 2, Walking Stick Press, 2003, 2009.

Hawken, P. The Magic of Findhorn, Bantam, 1982.

Hay, L. Heal Your Body, Hay House, 1984.

Hay, L. You Can Heal Your Life, Hay House, 1984.

Heinerman, Dr. J. Natural Pet Cures: Dog & Cat Care the Natural Way. Prentice Hall Press, 1998.

Hicks, E & J. The Amazing Power of Deliberate Intent, Hay House, 2006.

Holick PhD MD, M. The UV Advantage, IBooks Inc, 2005.

Hutchens, A. Indian Herbology of North America, Boston: Shambhala, 1973.

Integrative Medical Arts Group. Hepatotoxic Herbs. IBISmedical.com, 1998 –2000.

Jackson, A. The Ten Secrets of Abundant Health. Pendry Press, 2012.

Kaminski, P & Katz, R. Flower Essence Repertory: A Comprehensive Guide to North American and English

Flower Essences for Emotional and Spiritual Well-Being, Flower Essence Society, 1994.

Lad BAMS MASc, V. Ayurveda: A Brief Introduction and Guide. The Ayurvedic Institute, 2003.

Lee, MS et al. "Effects of external qi-therapy on emotions, electroencephalograms, and plasma cortisol". International Journal of Neuroscience, 2004 Nov;114(11):1493-502.

Lee, MS et al. "External Qi therapy to treat symptoms of Agent Orange Sequelae in Korean combat veterans of the Vietnam War." American Journal of Chinese Medicine, 2004;32(3):461-6.

Liberman, OD, PhD, J. Light: Medicine of the Future: How We Can Use It to Heal Ourselves NOW, Bear & Company, 1990.

Maclean, D. To Hear the Angels Sing, 1980.

Macrae, J. Therapeutic Touch: A Practical Guide, NY: Alfred A. Knopf, 1987.

Marshall Space Flight News Center, NASA. "Light emitting diodes bring relief to young cancer patients; NASA technology used for plant growth now in clinical trials." Accessed at http://www.nasa.gov/centers/marshall/news/news/releases/2003/03-199.html

Mayer MD, M. "Artificial Light Therapy in Tuberculosis." The Journal of the American Medical Association, June 14, 1924, Vol 82, No. 24.

McCulloch M, See C, Shu XJ, et al. Astragalus-based Chinese herbs and platinum-based chemotherapy for advanced non-small-cell lung cancer: meta-analysis of randomized trials. Journal of Clinical Oncology. 2006; 24:419-430.

McTaggert, L. The Field: The Quest for the Secret Field of the Universe. Harper Perennial, 2008.

Medical Economics. PDR (Physician's Desk Reference) for Herbal Medicine. Thomson Healthcare, 1998.

Meeus, C. Secrets of Shiatsu. Dorling Kindersley, 2000.

Melody. Love is in the Earth: A Kaleidoscope of Crystals - The Reference Book Describing the Metaphysical Properties of the Mineral Kingdom, Earth Lodve Publishing House, 1995.

Mercola, Dr. J. Emotional Freedom Technique: Basic Steps to Your Emotional Freedom, Accessed at eft.mercola.com, 2012.

Moon, H. Crystal Grids: How and Why They Work: A Science-Based, Yet Practical Guide, CreateSpace, 2001.

Monroe, R. Journeys Out of the Body, Broadway Books, 1992.

Monroe, R. Ultimate Journey, Three Rivers Press, 1996.

Motz, J. Hands of Life: From the Operating Room to Your Home, an Energy Healer Reveals the Secrets of Using Your Body's Own Energy Medicine. NY: Bantam, 1998.

Myss Ph.D., C. Anatomy of the Spirit: The Seven Stages of Power and Healing, Three Rivers Press, 1997.

National Center for Complimentary and Alternative Medicines: National Institutes of Health. http://nccam.nih.gov

Null Ph.D., G. The Complete Encyclopedia of Natural Healing.

Patterson, Dr. A. "Our Relationships With Light & Color." Accessed at http://www.inlightimes.com/archives/2001/02/color-light.htm

Rand, W.L. Reiki: The Healing Touch. Vision Publications, 1998.

Restoring the Earth: Visionary Solutions from the Bioneers. Tiburon, CA: HJKramer, Inc, 1997.

Rose, J. Herbs & Things. The Berkeley Publishing Group, 1972.

Schauss AG. "Tranquilizing effect of colour reduces aggressive behaviour and potential violence." J Orthomol Psych. 1979; 4:218–21.

Schiller, C. & Schiller D. 500 Formulas for Aromatherapy: Mixing Essential Oils for Every Use. Sterling Publishing, 1994.

Schnaubelt, K. Medical Aromatherapy. Frog Ltd., 1999.

Schoen, A.& Wynn, S.G.. Complementary and Alternative Veterinary Medicine: Principles and practice. NY: Mosby/Times Mirror. 1998.

Schoen, A. & Proctor, P. Love, Miracles, and Animal Healing: A Heartwarming look at the spiritual bond between animals and humans. NY: A Fireside Book/ Simon & Schuster, Inc. 1996.

Schoenbart L.Ac., B. Chinese Healing Secrets. Publications International, 1997.

Sigerist, H.E. A History of Medicine. Oxford University Press, 1951.

Silberman, S. "Placebos Are Getting More Effective. Drugmakers Want to Know Why." Wired Magazine, Issue 17.09.

Sills, F. The Polarity Process: Energy as a Healing Art, North Atlantic Books, 2001.

Simmons, R & Ahsian, N. The Book of Stones: Who They Are & What They Teach, North Atlantic Books, 2007.

Stein, D. Essential Reiki: A Complete Guide to an Ancient Healing Art. The Crossing Press, 1995.

Stojakowska A., Kadziaan B. & Kisiel W. Antimicrobial activity of 10-isobutyryloxy-8,9-epoxythymol isobutyrate. Fitoterapia, 2005: Volume 76, Issues 7-8, Pages 687-690.

Stone DO DC ND, Dr. Randolph, Polarity Therapy: The Complete Collected Works Volume 1 & 2. Book Publishing Company, 1999.

Tierra, L. The Herbs of Life: Health & Healing Using Western & Chinese Techniques. The Crossing Press, 1992.

Thai ND MSA, H.C. Traditional Vietnamese Medicine: Historical Perspective and Current Usage. 2003.

The Center for Reiki Research. Accessed at http://www.centerforreikiresearch.org.

"UV Light: Rediscovering the healing power of the sun," 2006, Minnesota Wellness Publications, Inc. Accessed at http://www.mnwelldir.org/docs/immune/ubi.htm

Von Muggenthaler, E. The Felid Purr: A Healing Mechanism. Fauna Communications Research Institute, 2001.

Wang, S.Y. and Zheng, W. "Antioxidant Activity and Phenolic Compounds in Selected Herbs". Journal of Agricultural and Food Chemistry, Vol. 49, No. 11: November, 2001.

Whelan, H. et al. "NASA Light Emitting Diode Medical Applications: From Deep Space to Deep Sea", A NASA study.

Wilcock, D. The Source Field Investigations. Dutton, 2011.

Wright, M.S. Behaving as if the God in All Life Mattered, Perelandra Ltd, 1997.

Love is in the Earth: A Kaleidoscope of Crystals - The Reference Book Describing the Metaphysical Properties of the Mineral KingdomWorwood, V. The Complete Book of Essential Oils and Aromatherapy. New World Library, 1991.

Yu MD, S. "Acupuncture and Acupuncture Meridian Assessment", Prevention and Healing.

Zukav, G. Dancing Wu Li Masters: An Overview of the New Physics. HarperOne, 2001.

About the Author

Maya Cointreau has over 18 years of experience in vibrational healing. She is an Usui Reiki Master and attuned in Karuna Reiki and the Iris Healing Method, along with having rigorously studied herbalism, polarity therapy, flower essences, traditional western naturopathy, homeopathy, crystal healing aromatherapy and shamanism. She co-owned and managed Hygeia, a holistic health and metaphysical wellness center for people in New Milford, CT, for five years and now runs Enchanted, a new age center, also in New Milford. Her previous books include "Grounding & Clearing," "Gesturing to God," "Natural Animal Healing," The Healing Properties of Flowers," "To the Temples" and "Equine Herbs & Healing."

Visit her author website at www.mayacointreau.com.

Other Books from
Earth Lodge Publications

Energy Healing for Animals & Their Owners: An Earth Lodge Guide to Pet Wellness

Sandra Cointreau

6x 9", 164 pages, B&W illustrations

Learn how to heal your animals with your own two hands. This informative book teaches animal communication and energy healing techniques, meditations and diagrams.

"Sandra Cointreau has written a very practical and easy to follow guide to the complex and subtle world of energy healing. Energy healing is something that those of us who love animals will want to learn and employ in our unending quest to make animals' lives better. Energy healing is a powerful tool, and Sandra shows you exactly how to use it." Marta Williams, Author/Animal Communicator, Learning Their Language and Beyond Words

"There are many different approaches and techniques that are collectively called Energy Healing therapies. This book describes approaches used in Energy Healing that may help animals recover from illness and injury and to maintain wellness." Allen M. Schoen, MS, DVM, Author, Kindred Spirits and Complementary and Alternative Veterinary Medicine

Natural Animal Healing: An Earth Lodge Guide to Pet Wellness

Maya Cointreau

6x 9", 160 pages, B&W illustrations

Natural Animal Healing includes natural health solutions for pets from many modalities including homeopathy, flower essences, energy healing, animal communications, aromatherapy, crystal healing, over 50 pages of herbs, a comprehensive table of ailments and corresponding remedies, and a multitude of gorgeous hand-drawn pen and ink illustrations.

Whether you have a cat, dog, or large animal this book offers informative, easy to follow guidance for pet wellness packed with enjoyable anecdotes and healing examples.

To The Temples: 14 Meditations for Healing & Guidance

By Maya Cointreau

6x 9", 130 pages, B&W illustrations

The beautifully guided meditations in **To The Temples** will take you to shrines and holy grounds that exist both in and out of this reality, places without time constraints, preconceived ideas or limitations. These inspiring meditations were designed by the author to help those on the path of healing, whether it be to heal oneself or to heal others. After each meditation you will find four blank, lined pages to record your thoughts.

Grounding & Clearing: Being Present in the New Age

Maya Cointreau

6x 9", 136 pages

Grounding & Clearing: Being Present in the New Age gives you the tools you need to remain a focused and empowered channel for your higher self, allowing you to manifest the reality you desire. We can only birth a better reality if we also remain grounded in the physical. In order to receive, embody and enact the messages that our higher selves send us, our bodies must be strong and aligned right along with our chakras and our souls. There is no mystery to the grounding techniques detailed in Grounding & Clearing. In this book you will learn techniques to ground in any situation, and to clear negative patterns and energies from your life. You will learn how to ground with prayer, scents, candles, symbols, colors, breath, nature, and more. With regular grounding and clearing, you will remain calm and focused while you free your spiritual gifts.

"For those just starting out on their spiritual journey and those "old timers" willing to take a little refresher course to brush up on some neglected business, I would like to recommend `Grounding & Clearing'. Every aspect of the subject matter is presented plainly and succinctly in a user friendly format designed to encourage as well as inform. While there is an abundance of books on a myriad of topics that claim to be a valuable resource one will go back to again and again, I believe this one really is. `Grounding & Clearing: Being Present in the New Age' will go a long way at helping to achieve that goal and point the way to that new reality." Brian Erland, Vine Voice Hall of Fame Reviewer.

Equine Herbs & Healing: An Earth Lodge Guide to Horse Wellness

By Maya Cointreau & E. Barrie Kavasch with Sandra Cointreau.

Foreword by Allen M. Schoen, MS, DVM

6x 9", 150 pages

The herbalists at Earth Lodge Herbals have brought together over 40 years of herbal experience to bring you this Earth Lodge Guide to Horse Wellness: Equine Herbs & Healing. This informative book teaches you how to combine and use herbs most effectively for your horse's benefit. Horses of the past were free to roam on large acreages and commonly sought out the native medicinal plants and herbs they needed to stay properly conditioned. Modern horses rely on their human owners to supply the herbs they need to keep their bodies strong and healthy. Learn what herbs have been used traditionally for which ailments and how to make your own salves, tinctures, braces, and sprays. The authors have included a handy reference table of disorders and their corresponding herbal remedies, as well as herbal recipes for the barn and home. Equine Herbs & Healing covers healing in many forms, from the historical uses of herbs to advances in aromatherapy and cancer therapy.

"Equine Herbs & Healing is a must-have resource." – Equine Wellness Magazine

"A great gift." – Natural Horse Magazine

Gesturing to God: Mudras for Physical, Spiritual & Mental Well-being

Maya Cointreau

Kindle Edition, 40 pages, 35 Full-Color illustrations

Mudras are symbolic hand gestures or positions used throughout the world in spiritual and daily practice. Studies show that they have the same effect on the brain as language: when you use a mudra, you are activating a specific thought or intent, and that thought carries energy, working like a radio signal to communicate with God, to All that IS, for fulfillment and manifestation. This book is a pocket guide to the mudras, illustrating over 35 mudras in a joyful and colorful way. Look at them when the mood strikes you, or use them every day. Above all: enjoy them!

Printed in Great Britain
by Amazon

48081668R00136

....

*** This book contains valuable and carefully researched information, but it is not intended to take the place of proper medical care and expertise. Please seek qualified professional care for health problems. ***

....

Cover Artwork, Layout & Design by Maya Cointreau